Hysteria

Hysteria has disappeared from contemporary culture only insofar as it has been subjected to a repression through the popular diagnosis of 'borderline personality disorder'.

In *Hysteria* the distinguished psychoanalyst Christopher Bollas offers an original and illuminating theory of hysteria that weaves its well-known features – repressed sexual ideas; indifference to conversion; over-identification with the other – into the hysteric form.

Through a rereading of Freud, Bollas argues that sexuality in itself is traumatic to all children, as it 'destroys' the relation to the mother, transfiguring her from 'mamma', the infant's caregiver, to 'mother', the child's and father's sex object. For the hysteric this recognition is endlessly traumatic and the hysterical personality forms itself into an organised opposition to this knowledge.

True to his earlier writings, Bollas' vision is thought provoking and mind expanding. *Hysteria* brings new perspectives to long-standing ideas, making enlightening reading for students and professionals involved in psychoanalysis and psychotherapy alike, as well as the lay reader who takes an interest in the formation of personality in western culture.

Christopher Bollas is a psychoanalyst in private practice in London. He is the author of *The Shadow of the Object* (1987), *Being a Character* (1992), *Cracking Up* (1995) *The New Informants* (with David Sundelson) (1995), and *The Mystery of Things* (1999).

Hysteria

Christopher Bollas

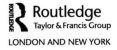

Routledge
Taylor & Francis Group

LONDON AND NEW YORK

First published in 2000 by Routledge
27 Church Road, Hove, East Sussex BN3 2FA

Simultaneously published in the USA and Canada
by Routledge
270 Madison Avenue, New York NY 10016

Routledge is an imprint of the Taylor & Francis Group, an Informa business

Reprinted 2000 (twice), 2002, 2006 and 2008

© 2000 Christopher Bollas

Typeset in Times by
Keystroke, Jacaranda Lodge, Wolverhampton
Printed and bound in Great Britain by
Biddles Ltd, King's Lynn, Norfolk

All rights reserved. No part of this book may be reprinted or
reproduced or utilised in any form or by any electronic,
mechanical, or other means, now known or hereafter
invented, including photocopying and recording, or in any
information storage or retrieval system, without permission in
writing from the publishers.

This publication has been produced with paper manufactured to strict
environmental standards and with pulp derived from sustainable forests.

British Library Cataloguing in Publication Data
A catalogue record for this book is available from the British Library

Library of Congress Cataloguing in Publication Data
Bollas, Christopher.
        Hysteria / Christopher Bollas.
            p.   cm.
        Includes bibliographical references and index.
        1. Hysteria.   1. Title.
    RC532.B64   1999   99–38081
    616.85′24—dc21   CIP

ISBN 978-0–415–22032–3 (hbk)
ISBN 978-0–415–22033–0 (pbk)

Contents

Introduction

His body imposes upon him a logic he detests. He replaces the body driven by its biology with an imaginary one symbolising his distress by enervating parts of it whilst showing little interest in its plight. He will be indifferent to it. Its sexuality seems divisive to him and, although he represses sexual ideas, paradoxically he finds they become rather powerful nuclei of the banished which continuously strive to return to consciousness. He will often dissociate himself from such returns, appearing cold and ascetic. Or he may do the opposite, becoming a kind of ringmaster to his internal world, exhibiting sexual ideas in his own ongoing theatre. Between these extremes he is lost in his own world of daydreams, where, amongst other possibilities, he can remain a perpetual innocent, living as a child inside the adult body. He can transmit his state of mind in adept ways, so much so that others of like temperament can identify with his plight. He could find himself in a community of kindred beings, all transmitting symptoms back and forth over their own psychic Internet.

He is an hysteric.

Any essay on hysteria is obliged to address its famous traits. When we think of hysteria we think of people who are troubled by their body's sexual demands and repress sexual ideas; who are indifferent to conversion; who are overidentified with the other; who express themselves in a theatrical manner; who daydream existence rather than engage it; and who prefer the illusion of childlike innocence to the worldliness of the adult. They also suffer from suggestion, either easily influenced by the other or in turn passing on ideas to fellow hysterics. Although others in the village of character disorders share one or more of the above traits, only the hysteric brings them together into a single dynamic form.

One task I have set myself is to provide a theory which weaves these traits into the hysteric form.

Theories of hysteria have tended to privilege certain perspectives at the expense of others, as if theories were small armies engaged in a war with one another. If one finds a biological contribution to the hysteric's interpretation of his or her plight – such as the hysteric's disenchantment with bio-logic's imposition of stages of sexual excitation – does this mean that the explanation rests on biology? If one addresses the hysteric's relation to the 'primary object' – initially, always the mother – does this mean that the theory rests on the self as derivative of maternal character? If one conceptualises the hysteric according to the dynamics of family life, does the theory stand or fall on the concept of family life?

In looking at something as complex as hysteria we are obliged to use as many perspectives as are necessary both to distinguish the essential traits and to forge them into an integrated vision of how each of these constituents influences, and is in turn affected by, the others. The reader will find that I give equal weight to the self's bio-logic, to its stages of psychic development, to its object relations, and to its formation in culture. My theory rests fundamentally on Freud's conceptualisation of hysteria – although there are areas where I disagree with him – but I have clearly been influenced in my thinking both by British object-relations theory – the schools of Klein and Winnicott – and by French psychoanalytic thought, especially the work of Lacan.

But on what basis do I construct my theory?

This book's strengths, and its limitations, are based on what I have been taught by my hysterical patients and by those hysterics whose treatments I have supervised. The reader will find that very often I discard theory in favour of an hysteric speaking for himself or herself; thus the book is full of clinical examples. The structure of the book is perhaps slightly unusual. A chapter may nominally be on the mother or on the father, yet only a part of the theory about the influence of each will be in that chapter. Further material on each will be found in other chapters, as will be true of all the themes in the work. There is, then, a certain repetition of the main concentrations – on sexuality, conversion, seduction, the mother, etc. – but the reader will find variations that introduce slightly different perspectives. The concerns of the text proceed rather in the manner of what Searle (p.2) calls 'criss-crossing continua', because it was first given in lecture form and the students needed to hear the main arguments repeated from time to time in order to follow them throughout the entire course of the seminar. I have elected to retain this format, not only because this is how it was originally composed, but also because I think the theory of hysteria is so complex that the reader will benefit from variegated recurrence.

The decision to deliver the lectures and subsequently to write the book derived from clinical supervisions in the USA in the mid-1980s. The cases being presented were clearly hysterics but the majority of the presenters thought of them as borderline personalities. Although in the past, supervisees had certainly presented a variety of character disorders, by the mid-1980s almost every case presented was hysteric. What was I to make of this? Gradually, it seemed to me to be an unconscious demand in the therapeutic community to reconsider hysteria. Disenchantment with the over-embracing concept of the borderline diagnosis was clear, and thinking the hysteric through the theoretical lenses of the borderline personality had become something of a tragedy.

I found myself giving micro-lectures on hysteria in the midst of supervisions, and then decided it was best to offer a seminar, which seemed to confirm the need to think this through. The ideas in this book were first presented at the Institute of

Contemporary Psychotherapy in New York in 1987 at the kind invitation of Edward Corrigan, which in turn led to two other seminars on hysteria in New York, one in 1991 and then again in 1996. I am grateful to the participants in these seminars for their critiques. The seminar was then presented in Chicago, São Paulo, Tel Aviv and Malmö and I wish to thank the psychoanalysts and psychotherapists in these communities for their comments, and especially those who provided many of the clinical vignettes to be found throughout this book.

In particular, I would like to thank Ulla and Lars Bejerholm, Gabriella Mann and Manoel Berlinck.

Chapter 1

The characters of psychoanalysis

Psychoanalytical case studies are for the most part discussions of human character and as we enter the new millennium the professional journals contain thousands of individuals described as suffering from one character disorder or another. Oddly enough, however, these essays do not describe human character, but failures in becoming a character true to one's potential.

How so?

Each self is born with an as yet unrealised idiom, which will partly come into its own true self through its use of those objects made available to it by parental care. If a self is comparatively free to establish its own idiom of being and relating through environmental provisions, then it will instantiate an idiosyncratic aesthetic, as it shapes and forms its world in a manner peculiar to itself. So each self will find particular individuals more attractive than others, will find certain actual objects – works of fiction, pieces of music, hobbies, recreational interests – of more interest than others, and in the course of living a life will have constructed a world which, although holding objects in common with other selves, will have shaped them into a form as unique as their fingerprint.

Character in itself is indescribable.

Psychoanalysis also distinguishes between a character state (such as a narcissistic state) and a character disorder (such as a narcissistic disorder), just as it differentiates all genres of conflict (schizoid, hysteric, etc.) from character disorders held under the same name. Placing any individual under one of these names recognises a structural fixation of what would otherwise simply be a character trait. All people move in and out of narcissistic states of mind, for example, when they are disinterested in the other's existence and are preoccupied with the self. As we shall discuss shortly, it is only when the person is consistently disinterested in the other that we begin to see if this trait now defines the self's fundamental relation to reality.

Are there mixed characters? Can someone be a narcissist, a borderline, a schizoid and an hysteric? Insofar as these define states of mind then a person can move into a narcissistic, a borderline, a schizoid or an hysteric frame of mind. Indeed, when we talk of a normal person, we are probably discussing anyone conflicted in such diverse ways that they are not under the spell of a fixation. Freud argued that any 'normal' person contains a polymorphous sexual history and still moves in and out of his or her infantile states of mind, to which Klein added that all people oscillate between paranoid-schizoid and depressive states of mind, or, as Bion maintained, between the psychotic and non-psychotic parts of the personality.

'Normal' means richly conflicted, or ill temporarily in so many ways that the self is free to articulate its form of being and relating. In the following chapters, however, when discussing the hysteric we are identifying someone's character fixation, and whenever we do this we identify a structural arrest that makes it difficult for someone to be a mixed character. As we shall see, a character disorder has taken a fundamental position in relation to its own primary object, which in the solipsism of fixation is a reflection of the self's partial arrest in being.

Psychoanalysts have many differing ways of discussing character disorders and each of the types I describe will be more of a cameo than an in-depth examination, as my aim here is to put the hysteric in the context of other disturbances of character. I shall limit myself to the fundamental object relation of each of these disorders, to the object which we shall call 'primary', and which calls for explanation.

When a person is disturbed his or her unconscious freedom is restricted and he or she is caught up in an unconscious relation to a primary object. It's as if the person were driving a car. When there are no problems, he or she is free to think about whatever crosses their mind, but if something starts going wrong with the car, the person's mind immediately focuses on the problem and their state of mind will become characteristic of dealing with that sort of problem in a particular sort of way.

But what is a primary object?

In a state of unconscious freedom the primary object is rather like a blank screen; it is anything we need or wish it to be in that moment – an open and useful space for the mental objectification of the passing wishes, memories, needs, reflections, plans and theories that are typical of moment-to-moment life. It rests upon the infant's experience of the good breast, something which, being there and being fulfilling, serves as the basis for the free imagining of selves and others. It is that introjected inner object that supports our thinkings and allows us all to be mental travellers articulating interests peculiar to our selves in the lived moments of everyday life.

However, when thrown into certain types of conflict, a troubling object emerges – even if unknown – and our unconscious freedom is immediately restricted by the redundant nature of the conflict. Borderline, schizoid and hysteric states refer to the structure of the self's conflict at any moment in time with a particular primary object.

What is the source of this primary object?

Its origins lie in the complex relation between infant and mother. If the good breast underwrites an object that is at our disposition to use as we wish, then the disturbing object is rather like a bad breast that provokes a different response. It is important to indicate what we discuss in the name of the mother.

When the mother is experienced as a bad object we are clearly not necessarily discussing the mother's character. In the first place, in the beginnings of life she is experienced less as an object than as a process which transforms the infant's physical, emotional and ideational life either positively or negatively. When she picks up and soothes the distressed infant she transforms the infant's inner state from distress to contentment. Alternatively, if she snatches a piece of cloth from the infant's mouth rather abruptly she can transform contentment into discontent.

As a process, however, she will be incorporated into the infant's system of self care, which is also an emerging process. Even if the developing child opposes maternal idioms of transformation, with a counter-process, something of the maternal process is betrayed in the child's selected alternative. These rules of engagement, procedures that become 'tacit assumptions'[1] about life and human relations, are not properly thought out by the infant and yet – taken in procedurally – become part of what is known. We might refer to these assumptions as 'unthought knowns' and we may see the evolution of a life, in part, as gradually realising the bases of one's unthought knowledge.[2]

Still, the informative effect of the maternal unconscious upon the infant's psychic life is profound. Heinz Lichtenstein argued that the mother 'imprints' an 'identity theme' (1961: 79) upon the infant, whilst Jean Laplanche writes that she is an 'enigmatic signifier' (1992: 21), whose unconscious life is so much more developed than the infant that her unconscious becomes an intrinsic part of the infant's own unconscious structure.

The Kleinian emphasis on the projective fate of the self's internal objects, put into the other through illocutionary acts that make of human speech a performative function, has always left open a door to a theory of the self's development according to the exchange of projective identifications between infant and mother. Kleinians have almost exclusively focused, however, on what the infant puts into the maternal container and how the mother receives, contains, transforms and communicates it back to the infant. But if we follow the path indicated by Lichtenstein and Laplanche – now elaborated according to the theory of projective identification – since the maternal unconscious is the more developed of the two, she will be projecting many ideas of her baby into the infant, both as an internal object (before conception, during pregnancy and through the many subtle shifting stages of childhood) and as her other, she will ultimately be projecting these ideas cumulatively through her own utterances and gestures as perfomances.

Freud did not examine human mental life from this very early perspective, but his concept of the 'thing presentation' more than allows for a link to be made to the maternal unconscious. The unconscious, according to Freud, is in the first instance made up of primary unconscious organisations, which are partly the outcome of the cumulative effect of the object world, a series of impressions of powerful objects that come to reside in the unconscious – as visual, kinaesthetic and sonic images – before the use of language. We may link Klein's theory of projective identification with Freud's theory of thing presentation, because what Freud means by a 'thing presentation' is in part the effect of maternal projective identification. As such, the infantile unconscious is populated by the maternal unconscious through constant acts of projective identification, which is not only ordinary, but essential to the work of breathing life into the infant. We may assume that if the mother's projections engage nascent developments of the infant's idiom, then her unconscious imaginatively elaborates the infant's self. In Chapter 3 we shall return to this topic when we consider maternal projective identification as a substitute for sensualised engagement with the infant.

When we speak of the primary object, however, we are not simply discussing the self's experience of the mother *per se*, although her way of being will be a vital contributing factor. The developing child also has his or her independent experience of the father and his idiom of transformation, and very possibly siblings, as well as early friends and their families. Indeed, he or she will be born into a family which is itself a complex of logical assumptions, which is larger than any one of its participants, and which goes relatively unexamined in the life of its members, even though the family mentality is a transformational object in its own right.

As Melanie Klein and her followers have stressed, the primary object will also be characterised by differing balances in the infant's economy of love and hate. An infant who, for genetic reasons, has a limited capacity to delay gratification will experience a mother as overly frustrating; this will increase the infant's hate toward the frustrating object and intensify the envy of the mother's breast, which is imagined to retain for itself what otherwise would be made available for the infant. We need not agree either with Klein's specific characterisations of the terms of this default in the infant or with the schedule in which she imagines it to appreciate the vital variable factor that includes the infant's subjective capabilities and disabilities as he or she negotiates with the object.

The primary object which we shall henceforth be referring to is a derivative of many experiences with actual others, some occasioned by environmental stresses – such as a hospitalisation, a move to a new home, a death in the family, parental divorce – some determined by character disorders of the mother and the father that are condensed into distressed experiences of the primary, and other factors having to do with the self's own constitutional liabilities.

A primary object, then, is determined by the self's psychic structure. Formed during the first years of life, this psychic structure projects the primary object that will be taken as the disposition of all others toward the self. In non-conflictual moments it may be benign, but when the self is disturbed it will reflect the structure of the self's pathology.

In discussing different character disorders, I am, for heuristic purposes, forced to simplify. So, in discussing distress with the primary object in terms of a problem with the mother, the reader should bear in mind what I mean by the mother, or what is held in her name: though it may well describe a true feature of her mothering, it will also include environmental factors disturbing the infant, as well as the infant's projection of his or her own circumstances on to the mother.

If the father is to be held responsible for the self's negotiated acceptance of the necessity to internalise and adhere to the laws of society, the mother is to be held responsible for the self's experience of existence itself. And just as for every failure of the child's father to uphold his role, we will find dynamic motivations in the child to destroy his function, so too with the mother: for every actual failure in her provision of care, we will find the infant self deforming her out of anxiety, rage or depression. We are left, then, when referring to the father or the mother to these figures as psychic structures. They shall always reflect the work of at least three people (child, mother, father) and the internal object that emerges is the self's experience of 'the world', a formation whose primacy underwrites being and relating.

As such, all the character disorders can partly be understood as an adjustment made in relation to the mother. Whether referring to the psychotic, the borderline or the neurotic character, we are in the first place describing a restriction of the self bound up with anxieties in relation to the mother.

Let us begin with the narcissistic disorder.

Experiencing the mother as uneven, the infant resolves the problem she poses by eradicating her and putting a part of the self in her place. This is the classic narcissistic pose: apparent infatuation with the self. Irrespective of whether the infant puts an idealised part of the mother or some other in place of the truly different mother, the narcissistic strategy is to replace the other with some harmonic object that will support the narcissist's search for tranquillity.[3] In their disturbed relations narcissists will search for someone to idealise them, thus finding in this other someone compatible with their own self love. All will go fruitfully until such time as the other disagrees. It is not simply that the narcissist finds difference with the self difficult to take, but difference in itself is hard to bear. Indeed, the narcissist's strategy is largely aimed at oblating differences between self and other, seeking relations with common objects around which idealisation may occur.

Inclined towards harmony, narcissists are disinclined to entertain the complexities of lived experience, as this predisposes them to encountering difference. Thus they will seek less complex internal issues and try to pursue a life relatively free of the unwanted or undesirable. As this may incline them towards being rather boring, they will often seek a partner who is lively and interesting, but not a challenge to their self-esteem because they are the object of idealisation. So they can piggyback on the other's interest in life and gain nutrition through the other's bearing of the inevitable conflicts that come with encountering difference.

In psychoanalysis such patients often idealise the analyst in an unconscious effort to have the analyst return this type of love in the form of empathic mirroring,[4] but they are liable to states of rage and distress when they feel judged or criticised. At such moments they may obliterate what difference exists in the analyst's way of thinking. In the extreme, if they cannot restore their harmony through self idealisation they may experience a psychic vacuum created by annihilation of the maternal object of difference. This will precipitate a narcissistic depression, which they believe can only be relieved through a powerful act of transforming love, one which is so intoxicating that all memory of the acts of annihilation, of the vacuum and of the murderous self are eliminated from consciousness.

Narcissistic states of rage, commonly regarded as a typical feature of the narcissistic personality, are more like anxiety attacks that abreact panic through a rage intended to restore harmony. Although an unconscious violent action has removed differentiated otherness from view, ironically, narcissists lack generative aggression. They are disinclined to struggle – to put the self or their ideas forward, since struggle implies difference – which leads them to take refuge in a semi-fortified Arcadian world of self objects.

Psychoanalysts frequently experience narcissistic patients as initially appealing and charming, but eventually as uninteresting and boring, causing the analyst to feel sleepy during sessions. The narcissist will often negatively hallucinate the analyst's interpretive work, continuing to talk as if the analyst had not spoken, and the analyst often struggles to exist as a meaningfully separate object.

The borderline person is different. He or she has experienced the primary object as causing so much turbulence to the self that inner states of mental turmoil have become equivalent to it.[5] To simplify: it is as if the infant has experienced a rhythmic mothering, being physically or psychically picked up in disruptive ways, evoking a mixture of shock, anxiety, rage, a type of loss and intense mentation all in one which is associated with the mother. The solution to what would seem to be a most distressing state of affairs is to split the object and to construct an ideal object – stitched together out of bits of the good mother – as a fragile alternative to the other mother. Unfortunately, this solution is always a temporary one, because the borderline feels that his or her core object is to be found only through turbulent states of mind. Unconsciously, therefore, the borderline character seeks out turbulence, turning molehills into mountains, and escalating irritations into global states of rage. Evolved 'whole objects', acquired through cognitive development, are tertiary to the primary object, which exists only in the fragmented state described above.

In the transference they will split the analyst, between a fragile idealised object and a denigrated object that feels more true, more primary. When seeking this split object they will exploit errors of analytical interpretation or other failures on the analyst's part, converting such mistakes into paranoid feeding festivals, the strange delight disguised by the intensity of mental anguish. In the counter-transference, analysts working with such patients feel anxious, frustrated, often irritated, sometimes angry and ill at ease.

The schizoid character finds the mother only intrusive, but rather than oblate the difference of the object, like the narcissist, or subsume the self into the affective cocktail produced by the actions of the object, like the borderline, the schizoid stands back and says something like 'What is going on here? Who is this other? And who am I?' The schizoid turns the relational space into something of a laboratory where the self becomes a research scientist. In their researches they populate the mind with a thousand different mothers, fathers and selves. Each intense experience of a life is repeatedly examined in the mind until gradually the mind becomes that fundamental object of dependence. Contemplating future experiences, the schizoid thinks them out in advance – considering all the possible options – so that such thinking eventually substitutes for experience itself.

In the transference the schizoid seeks to use the mind – with its associative potentials – as an end in itself. The schizoid wants to talk and explain his or her inner world to the analyst, and dreads emotional experience as it usually brings closer a form of surrender to the primary object, which, for the schizoid, it is preferable to keep at a distance. He or she often evokes countertransferences in which the analyst is fascinated with the schizoid's inner life, so much so that the analyst is actually lulled into a kind of schizoid state, in which the mind as an object is accepted as an end in its own right. The clinical innovations of Winnicott, Balint and Khan, amongst others, were directly aimed at finding techniques within psychoanalysis that did not collude with the schizoid use of analytical interpretation.

Right away we may see important differences among these different characters.

The narcissist seeks to sustain an empty self, whilst the schizoid is full of objects. The borderline seeks out turbulent mental states, whilst the narcissist rages in order to retain harmony. The schizoid experiences emotional life as bringing closer an uneasy surrender to the primary object and thus prefers emotional aloofness, whilst the borderline seeks emotionally enmeshing encounters.

The pervert is the character most often compared to the hysteric. Freud played with the idea that they were inversions of one another, and in the 'Three Essays . . .' (1905) it was the pervert that he used as the comparative benchmark for the hysteric. On the surface, they seem strikingly different in one respect: the hysteric represses sexual contents whilst the pervert acts them out. Both characters, however, privilege sexuality as problematic. Both operate in a kind of dissociated auto-erotic state, and the pervert cruising for the object of desire and the hysteric daydreaming it may collide in the street in separate worlds of sexual preoccupation. In the final chapter, we shall return to some of the similarities and differences, but what can be said now about the pervert's relation to the primary object?

Perverts are compelled, against their conscious volition, to imagine or act out a particular erotic scene that dominates the entirety of their sexual existence. They attempt to reverse this subjugation, by portraying themselves as master of the instincts, presuming to be in charge of a situation beyond their control. Loss of the illusion of dominance leaves them feeling close to a sense of personal annihilation, as if their existence had to proceed according to this illusion. What psychoanalysts believe can be seen in the complex structure of perversion is the self's effort to recover from a sexually exciting other – experienced as the mother – who nearly brought the self to a state of psychic extinction. This is a mother whose fundamental cathexis of the infant is as her secret sex object, which she acts out in emotionally detached scenes of excitation discharge, using the child as her fantasy object. Whilst the mother of the hysteric retreats into her imaginary universe, there to create a sexual relation to a purely internal object, the mother of the pervert acts this out in the real. This may be a reflection of the mother's character, or equally of her circumstances at that time of her life. She could be emotionally removed from her infant because of a post-partum depression, or a loss in the family, or a disturbing move, or any of innumerable reasons.

The pervert as infant, then, experiences his or her sexuality as attacking from the real, as approaching not through the intrapyshic channels of the psychic economy of the infant's own instincts – seeking to join internal object with actual others over time – but careening into him or her without psychic notice.

To think now of the pervert as child, this excitation is fragmenting, as the self and its other seem to have bits of relation to one another, but not brought together. As the self's excitation is itself part of the disintegrating experience, the pervert then aims to reorganise his or her predicament by putting himself or herself in charge; as an adult the pervert must find others willing to be put through the perverse exchange. The compulsive sexuality of the pervert is in fact a device to rid the self of the alienating consequences of instincts provoked by the other; the pervert seeks to disrupt the other by projectively identifying the entire complex into a victim. Perverse communities form in order to divide the roles – some conquering for the moment, others performing the vanquished – and find new forms of intimacy within the sexual universe, given that it has always been the venue of alienation.

The pervert's primary object is his or her instinct-object, which the pervert is compelled to seek, often against his or her conscious wishes. The instinct-object is to be found in the other, who, as a like subject, is also driven to an instinct-object that alienates the self from its desire. When the pervert meets his or her opposite the pervert finds *only* sexual-discharge intimacy that echoes the early experience of being the other's instinct-object and nothing else. As we shall see, the pervert shares something of the hysteric's conviction that his or her sexual destiny resides in the other's imaginary; but the pervert has been actively used as the mother's object of quick excitation – which the pervert marries to his or her own instinct experience – whilst the hysteric has experienced the withdrawal of maternal excitation, which he or she seeks out in the mother's internal world, where it is assumed to exist in purely auto-erotic form.

We could proceed through the entire characterology of psychoanalytic figures and consider each one of them according to its primary object relation, but the cameos of each character above are intended only to give the reader a sense of what is meant by the primary object relation, in order to study hysteria more completely. In the following chapters we shall consider the many different sides to the hysteric, in many respects the most complex character of all.

I will begin our study of the hysteric by constructing a *modelo* comparable with those of the narcissist, the borderline and the schizoid characters. With the exception of the 'malignant hysteric' (see Chapter 11), the hysteric's relation to the primary object differs from those of the other character disorders. In most instances, the hysteric witnesses intense, if detached, maternal love of the self, evidenced by maternal narrative passion about the child and/or maternal performance of her love in the presence of the child. What is missing, as we shall see, is an unconscious sense of maternal desire for the child's sexual body – especially the genitals – but in other respects the child often experiences maternal interest, passion, investment and care. The mother is in conflict over her child, whom she knows she has failed. In the presence of this primary object, the child seeks out who he or she is to the mother and then tries to identify with this object of desire and to represent it to the mother. The hysteric's ailment, then, is to suspend the self's idiom in order to fulfil the primary object's desire, a strategy based upon the complementary actions of identification and representation.

Consideration of the hysteric requires a particular theory of maternal character. At times it will seem as if her mentality determines the fate of her infant. The idea that the primary object is a psychic creation of the child will seem to be discarded by the theory of the mother who is herself hysteric.

This understanding would be partly correct. Ironically, because this mother has been successful in supporting her infant, the infant's underlying sense of being is not jeopardised, certainly not as it is with the borderline, schizoid or narcissistic personality. The self's primary object in these more psychotic disturbances is a collage of fragments, a collection of part objects. Not only is the hysteric's object a whole object, supplying a coherent sense of itself, but the hysteric possesses a unique capacity to identify with complex aspects of the other's character, an ability that testifies to the mother's skill in developing her infant's sense of self and other. In one single respect, in her sexuality, she is insecure and this she communicates to her infant. In this alone, we decide that the hysteric's mother has made her own distinctive contribution to her infant.

Because the mother has supported the hysteric's being, however, the hysteric's primary object will be any other into whom the hysteric is projected and through whom an identity is to be selected for acting out. In conflictual states this means that the hysteric's primary object will be the object-in-waiting that the hysteric must find in order to be recast as the other's object of desire. In conflict, the hysteric is already filling out this object through acting out, even if the other from whom the object is extracted is still unknown.

Let us now turn to the heart of the matter: the hysteric's disaffection with his or her sexual life.

Notes

1   See Michael Polanyi, *On Tacit Knowledge*.
2   For a discussion of the concept of the 'unthought known' see my *Shadow of the Object* (Bollas, 1985).
3   See Herbert Rosenfeld's work, *Impasse and Interpretation* (1987).
4   See Heinz Kohut's analysis of narcissism in *The Analysis of the Self* (1971).
5   See my essay 'Borderline desire', in *The Mystery of Things* (Bollas, 1999).

Chapter 2

Sexual epiphany

Around 3 years of age children experience a meaningful intensification in sexual excitement, as biological maturation drives newly intense genital sexual sensations. They masturbate more frequently and with more acuity. By touching the penis or the clitoris, respectively, boys and girls create rather blissful sensual states.

Like Freud's 'Little Hans' they may quite naturally invite the parents to do the same. At 4¼, while being bathed by his mother, who powders around his penis – 'taking care not to touch it' – Hans asks, 'Why don't you put your finger there?' The conversation proceeds:

> *Mother*: 'Because that'd be piggish.'
> *Hans*: 'What's that? Piggish? Why?'
> *Mother*: 'Because it's not proper.'
> *Hans*: 'But it's great fun.'

(Freud, 1909: 19)

Another of Hans's contemporaries would have agreed with him. Freud tells of a patient putting on her daughter's 'drawers', and 'to do this she passed her hand upwards along the inner surface of the child's thigh. Suddenly the little girl shut her legs together on her mother's hand, saying: "Oh, Mummy, *do* leave your hand there. It feels so lovely"' (ibid., p. 19).

With this new sexual intensity come different mental representations as the child imagines the mother's and the father's body in more distinctly sexual terms.

The mind is more fully occupied by sexuality.

Boys and girls act on this new excitement by seeking out the mother's genitals, by direct request or by 'accident'. Depending on the mother, such penetrations (as well as poking her breasts, probing her bottom, locking legs around a part of her body) may be occasions of delight or annoyance. In time, such intercourses become discomforting and the parents refuse the child's foreplay.

Although Freud tended to emphasise the boy's love relation with the mother – 'When a boy (from the age of two or three) has entered the phallic phase of his libidinal development, is feeling pleasurable sensations in his sexual organ and has learnt to procure these at will by manual stimulation, he becomes his mother's lover' (1940: 189) – he saw both boys and girls as engaged in a 'masculine' love relation to the mother.

All children find this change disturbing. In a sense, the former relation to the mother is destroyed by a new set of mental representations. Although the infant–mother relation is erotic right from the beginning, transformation of the mother-as-comforter into the mother-as-sex-object breaks up a particular sense of her as a sensual provider, almost a part of the self's auto-erotic universe. She is distinctively different because her body is now seen more precisely as the object of sexual desire, and sexuality-in-itself changes the child's life forever. It is ironic that this epiphany at around 3 actually organises the infant's and the mother's prior erotic relations to one another, something to which we will return later.

This shift in the mother's status is caused by the change in the child's libido, which is no different with the girl than with the boy, as both children experience sexuality as revolutionary.

So, sexuality destroys the innocence of a self and mother, transforming the prelapsarian utopia of 'baba' and 'mama' into the world of self and sex object, contaminating the simplicity of dependence with desire. There is no original sense of innocence, it is only conceived after original sin. In the wake of genital excitation the self invents innocence, usually removing it from the present, where it can be sullied by the everyday and putting it into the past, where it may be more easily enshrined.

Certain memories of sexual abuse recall the moment when sexuality intruded upon the self. 'I have learned to explain a number of phantasies of seduction', writes Freud in 1906, 'as attempts at fending off memories of the subject's *own* sexual activity (infantile masturbation)' (1906: 274). In 'The aetiology of hysteria' (1896) Freud writes that 'an attempted rape perhaps, reveals to the immature girl at a blow all the brutality of sexual desire' (pp. 200–1), implicitly arguing that rape signifies the brutality of sexuality and not simply the act of a brutal man.

Sexuality-in-itself, intensified, as we shall discuss later at some length, by the child's auto-erotic stimulations, is the agency of trauma, all by its fearsome self.

Seeing the mother as sexual is not a supplement to the mother created by oral and anal excitations. The pre-genital is in a different category, in exactly the way that Gilbert Ryle (1963) argues that the separate buildings of a university and what the term 'university' names are in different categories. In Ryle's famous example, a man asks to be directed to the university, but after seeing all the buildings asks again where to find the university. He has not realised that the university is in a separate category from the buildings he has seen and that he is asking the wrong question. At 3 the child discovers sexuality and perceives the mother in a different light. Her sexual dimensions had always existed before this epiphany, just as the buildings of the university existed, but it takes a different categorical realisation suddenly to see the sexual mother. Sometime later the child will see the mother or the father at work and perceive them according to the newly discovered category of wage-earner.

We may now rethink the well-known conundrum posed by Freud. The hysteric suffers from a 'scene of seduction', first understood by Freud to be at the hands of one of the parents, later to be understood as driven by the child's fantasy life. The scene of seduction, however, is the disruptive arrival of sexuality-in-itself driven by the child's bio-logic. As we shall see in subsequent chapters, the parents have all along been engaged in an intense seduction of the child, teasing him or her from the child's auto-erotic cocoon *into* passionate sexual love of the other. The scene of seduction is a true crossroads between the self's sexual drive and the other's seduction.

Sexuality and death are linked by this epiphany, as a certain image of a solely comforting mother dies. The child must now survive his or her imagining of the mother's desire, driven by merciless instinctual states that promote sexual consciousness. For Freud the maternal vagina is horrifying because it forces the child to confront his anxiety over castration, but, even if we allow some truth to this idea, it also announces the elemental shock that mum is now gone forever, signifying the death of infancy, the first of many deaths that affect each self from within the real.

As sexuality is the genesis of a rift in the self, it is not surprising that it draws to it like a magnet all the issues surrounding this first death – most famously, the association of orgasm with death. This epiphany forges links between a non-verbal and a verbal arrival, between the movement of the body in erotic states and the imagining of the body and its other in fantasy, between the urge that is the instinct and its mental representations on the border of the biological and the cultural. Questions that surround sexuality – not the least being 'What is it?' – are simply parts of the original complex imposed upon the child. What is happening to the self? How is one to understand this development?

Kohon's (1986) important essay stresses the hysteric's impossible position, stuck between two objects of desire (mother and father), unable to go from one to the other. Part of the limbo is the outcome of this sexual epiphany, when the child is suddenly aware of two mothers, two fathers and two selves at the very least: pre-genital and genital. The question of who one desires cannot be easily answered by the hysteric, unsure of what he or she wishes.

All children seek temporary refuge from this conflict, as it is impossible to acknowledge that one's sexuality is the agent of this change. Comfort is sought by putting it outside the mother–child relation, inevitably pointing to the third object, the father. 'He did it! He is to blame for this disruption!' If the father is 'good enough' he will accept this projection and bear it with patience, as he knows that however much he is lovingly included in the infant's world, other parts of him are unwanted and hated. Assigned an important function – to bear the child's hate of the outside world and all that it augurs – the father's task is to accept the projected. (It is of interest that this projection of excitation returns later in the identification of sexuality with the father – part of why the girl finds him sexy and the boy finds him a ready-made object of sexual destiny. All the while, the father will carry repressed excitement to be returned later by the irony of an identification that is in fact a reclamation. A similar projection has occurred in relation to the mother, as each child projects nurturing and caretaking feelings into her, so that, much later, when looking after the other, the self enjoys a narcissistic return of early projections.)

To gain an early sense of both our similarity with and our difference from the hysteric, it is important to see that in the unconscious life of any person – male or female – there is a fantasy of having been molested by the father. This is an important consideration, given the mayhem created by indiscriminate beliefs in the patients' accounts of 'recovered memories' of sexual abuse. The molestation, however, is sexuality itself, which breaks the relation to the mother and transforms the bliss of ignorance into the sin of sexual knowledge. The father is 'sexuality-as-trauma', a molesting figure whose sexuality drives a wedge between child and mother, forever problematising the child's sense of goodness.

What had been Edenesque is now ruined by the serpent, which drives God the mother to abandon us to our fate.

In 1852, when she was 'journeying' across the country speaking against slavery and for women's rights, the black American activist Sojourner Truth met up with a cleric at an equal rights convention who opposed greater inclusion of women in society. The activist said: 'That little man in black there, he says women can't have the same rights as men, because Christ wasn't a woman! Where did your Christ come from? From God and a woman! Men had nothing to do with him.'[1] Turning the core hysteria of Christianity on its head – as the theology not only excludes sexuality from the relations of the deity to His, or more correctly Her, creations, but subsequently sees carnality as the ongoing foe of devotion to Her – Sojourner Truth cannily capitalised on the vigorous exclusion of the sexual father from an intercourse that must be immaculate.

The sexual father does have his uses, however, especially as the villain meant to bear evil. In the current epidemic of hysteria in the North American world, the father is continuously used to protect the individual from the unsavoury effects of sexual states of mind, as the self and its innocents simply need protection from sexually predatory men cruising the world looking for more child victims to satisfy sexual cravings.

Upon realisation of one's sexuality, projected into the father and then repudiated, the sexual father is castrated – either marginalised for a while or removed entirely, as in Christian theology. Although a part of the superego that arrives as a critical agency, inflicting internal prohibitions – and making threats – is an internalisation of the forbidding father, the young child's mind also develops its critical sense from disapproval of the emergence of sexuality itself, which disrupts the graceful privilege of the infant–mother couple. This agency of investigation – sponsoring questions such as 'What is going on here?', 'Who is really in charge here?', etc. – filtrates into the superego, which then proceeds to commit forms of violence against the father. So much so that paternal enmity will be energised by the child's violent refusals of the father's reality and his sexual function.

Freud's theory of the castration complex includes early castrations (i.e. weaning, toilet training, etc.), to which we add the castration of sexuality itself. The father becomes the sign of this intrusion and is irreversibly associated with sexuality as the unwanted.

Castration anxiety proper – the fear of genital mutilation – does not entirely spring from the consequence of imagined incestuous urges but also from the self's attack upon its own genitals and those of the other.

As it is very hard to recall the sexual epiphany of 3, fortunately we have another scene that recapitulates it in many ways. Most people recall what it felt like to have been 7, 8 or 9. Sexual states of mind existed, but the world of boys and girls, intense good friendships, school life, after-school play and holidays seemed somehow idyllic. Then sometime around 10 – earlier for some, later for others – bodies start changing again. With the changing shape of the body, which – however anticipated and partly welcomed – is to some extent disconcerting, comes another increase in sexual excitation. The adolescent feels assaulted by sexual ideas. Sitting in a classroom with childhood friends of old, suddenly a 13-year-old is deeply excited by another student, and finds it very hard to think about the lesson. That other student need not be in the classroom. The instinct is provocation enough for the adolescent to feel its disruptiveness whilst furtively daydreaming his or her sex objects.

Blissful as this is, it is also disruptive. For one thing, adolescents feel that childhood friendships will never be the same again. There may be a kind of retrospective idealisation of pre-adolescent years, highlighting the turmoil of adolescence even more. Parents' bodies are once again seen as more intensely sexual presences and, although many adolescents will almost leap with relief upon bodily imperfections of the parent, they do so because these sexually exciting bodies are just too much to bear.

Once again this disruption may be projected into another figure. It may be the father seen as sexually dangerous, a projective identification that testifies to the child's difficulty in accepting his or her own bodily excitations. Customarily, however, adolescents establish sexual ideals – figures in the music world or cinema, for example – who contain the self's sexuality, allowing more time to contain the alienating aspects of sexual life. As time passes the adolescent nominates new sex objects and casts off old ones, eventually engaging in sexual relations with peers, which, amongst other things, allow greater familiarity as the owner-operator of the body engine.

If the memory of adolescence feels too dim to be fruitfully stirred, perhaps this account by a patient will bring the point home.

> I was at a business meeting last week and there were the same old faces, really, and we were meant to come up with our final report, which as you know is very important this time of year, when this new bloke – Eddie, who has been there for about three weeks – well, when I realised I was looking at him more than . . . well . . . you see . . . the fact is that I was suddenly amazingly turned

on by the sight and presence of him. I couldn't think. And when at a certain point the boss asked me what I thought I flushed red in the face and although it's completely ridiculous I thought that everyone must know what I was going through. Of course they didn't, although I said I wasn't feeling well. But as time passed it all got worse and my heart was racing . . . and other things were happening . . . and it was all I could do to get out of the room. I could curse that man. Until he arrived, this was a wonderful place just to get to work on our tasks, and now he has gone and fucked it all up.

With this fast-forward into adolescence and adult life, we may return to the 3-year-old, who has undergone a similar biological shock, but who is much less capable than the adolescent of processing sexuality. Although it would be foolhardy to try to deconstruct the ingredients of sexual attraction, one of its consequences is to leave any self arrestingly aware of bodies and their drives – a crucial factor in thinking of the hysteric, who is most deeply at odds with the body which drives the self to consider mental contents, thereby ruining the self's desire for simplicity and innocence.

Before moving on, however, we need to dwell for a moment on the irony of a movement within this chapter itself. To explain the effect of bio-logic on the 3-year-old I have deferred it to adolescence, where it is easier for us to recall the impact of the self's sexual life. In fact, I have followed the path of the child's *Nachträglichkeit* ('deferred action'). Unable to think to themselves the effect of their sexuality, because they are too psychically immature, children defer its meaning for later. With adolescence there is a second occurrence of the force of sexuality upon the self, and it is at this moment that the self will be capable of rethinking the trauma of sexuality.

The 3-year-old represses aspects of the meaning of his or her sexual life, deferring them until much later, when subsequent lived experiences will combine to facilitate de-repressions of the infantile experience of genital sexuality. Nonetheless, the child of 3 is *on the verge* of discovering just how complex he or she is.

Indeed, with the partial realisation of the self's sexual mental contents, the child interpolates the mother's sexuality. She is no longer simply mum-the-provider, she is also now the mother who desires, and in particular – ordinarily – the mother who desires the father. The comforting illusion that mummy and daddy came together in order to bring a child into existence is now dispelled. Apart from Jesus (or 'the Holy Family'), the child did not enter existence through maternal immaculate conception. There was an intercourse. On the one hand, this actuates a narcissistic crisis, since the child is not only not the centre of the universe, but possibly an after-effect of parental sexual passion sought after for its own sake. This news is not transmitted by parental instructions about the nature of sexuality – although that may happen in certain families – nor even by the occasional sight of the parents in bed, nor of animals engaged in intercourse. Children supply the idea of parents coming together for sexual passion from the biological fact of their own auto-erotic adventures. They have their fingers up their vagina, or their hands on their penis, and explore their anus a good part of every week. They are driven to their theories of adult sexual passion by their own bodies, and they imagine intercourse in terms of their own infantile preoccupations.

Being embodied is a mixed fate for the hysteric, who does not want to be excluded by anyone from anything, and yet, given the shocking secrets of sexuality – revealed by the self's own developing body knowledge – experiences this body and what it knows as a depraved epistemology. This fact is a vital constituent in the formation of the hysteric because in so many differing ways – enervation in the nineteenth century, fatigue in the twentieth century – hysterics indicate trouble with the body. It imposes the unwanted, and the response to the body's invasion of the self varies from irritated indifference to paranoid grudge.

The child's psychic realisation of the contextual meaning of sexuality is humbling. To discover that maternal desire is not restricted to the wish for this infant, and that the mother and the father have independent sexual wishes, seems an attack upon the visions of the self as the centre of the parental universe.

Inside this new state of affairs children start asking questions. Typically, they want to know where they were before they were born. When given an answer they are very often struck by the existential questions that arise. Where do we all come from, then? Where were mum and dad before they met? How did they meet? Where were grandma and grandpa? Where is God? What happens after we die? Where is heaven? This moment in a young child's life initiates an intense period of questioning about . . . everything. However much it exhausts parents, the fact that the parent supplies an answer, establishes the mother and the father in the place of – to use Lacan – the one who is supposed to know. Through these answers the child is given complex sets of directions. If the child chooses to follow them, then he or she will grow up in the image of the gender that is supplied by these answers and many more. In other words, out of the crisis of the 3-year-old self, a child moves into the oedipal period already predisposed towards certain identifications.

Freud postulates that any self's search for knowledge is driven by the anxiety that arrives upon the child's recognition of sexual difference. The question 'Where is the penis?', asked by the child upon sight of the female genital, is the mother of all questions and the genesis of the search for all knowledge. The child hysteric will develop a learning disorder of sorts, as he or she will deal with this aspect of sexuality's disruptive presence by creating gaps in what he or she knows.

How many children identified as 'attention deficit disorders' or as 'dyslexic' are hysterics who eject knowledge rather than learn or who unconsciously sabotage cognitive development? The hysterical boy or girl is proclaiming an innocence of knowledge in order to assert his or her pre-sexual relation to the mother. He or she attacks cognitive development by disabling the self's maturation, always symbolically celebrating the position of the innocent child.

Normal children accept the powerful logic of their own development. 'I am forced into realisation by my excitements' transforms into: 'I find you [mum] exciting', transforms into: 'I find your excitements exciting', transforms into: 'I shall identify with your sexuality', transforms into: 'we are all in this together'. Thus the loss of virginal love is softened by desire operating through acts of identification which feel sexual and progressive at the same time. The boys' 'I want mummy' and the girls' 'I want daddy' are erotic transformations of primary desire, in which identification with the primal scene elicits and directs sexual life.

The realisation that one has been pushed out by the father is transformed by identification ('I shall now choose parental objects of desire'), so that the child's hate may now be fused with his or her sexuality. In a few years, the child transforms loss, impotence and innocence into the theatre of sexual choice.

The self will marry the parent of the opposite sex and bring forth new children, making mummy and daddy, and grandma and grandpa, very happy. Not to mention the clerics, schoolteachers and custodians of small-child culture.

But the hysteric does not rest easy with the problematics of his or her own sexuality and even less with the ordinations that emerge from this initiation. For reasons which will be discussed in the following two chapters, the hysteric resists going forward.

Following the projection of sexuality-as-molestation into the father, the hysteric seeks a return to the mother through a desexualisation of the self and of the mother, whilst the non-hysteric progresses through a sexualisation of self and other. The desexualisation is usually accomplished through idealisation of the mother's non-sexual characteristics – turning her into a Madonna and the self into a sexual innocent. Aiming to be another's perfect little girl or perfect little boy, the hysteric energises idealisation through libido-as-desexualisation. The father may also be included in this constellation through a similar act of splitting, where as the bad sexual father he is either repressed or projected into a known bad sexual man – such as a child-molester on TV – just as the sexual mother has been split off into the bad sexual woman – such as a recognised slut.

The 'good-enough' hysteric constructs an ideal self and an ideal mother who repudiate sexuality as divisive. The internal mother disapproves of sexuality and wishes the hysteric to remain her child forever. Sexuality must be found disgusting. (The taste metaphor trades on the oral relation to the mother's body, leading the self to spit out the genital experience through identification and projection.) The 'death-drive' hysteric (to be discussed in detail later) constructs a cold mother violently opposed to the self's manifestation of the sexual and this child assumes a frigid goodness.

The hysteric's ego ideal will be an internal mirror of the perfect self. 'The ego ideal is now the target of the self-love which was engaged in childhood by the actual ego' writes Freud in 'On narcissism' (1914). 'The subject's narcissism', he continues, 'makes its appearance displaced on to this new ideal ego, which, like the infantile ego finds itself possessed by every perfection that is of value.' He concludes: 'what he projects before him as his ideal is the substitute for the lost narcissism of his childhood in which he was his own ideal' (ibid., p. 94). Freud's essay is on the self's normal development, and to this extent one may find an ordinary hysteria in the self's construction of its ideal self. The child who will become hysteric will sustain a rigidly pure ideal that specifically targets its sexual life as degrading, and will seek to transcend such contamination by continually asserting the presence of an ideal self through testimonial good behaviour or ascetic removal from all relations.

Masud Khan (1983) saw in the development of the hysterical child a false self, and it is easy enough to see how, through eradication of the child's own instincts, sexual passions are transformed into the ecstasy of self-sacrifice, in which instincts are given up for presumed love by the mother and the father. This sacrifice is not only culturally supported, but is also the object of a certain parental and social adoration.

This attempt at desexualisation puts the hysteric in direct conflict with his or her own sexual body. At a crucial moment in the life of the child in which his or her genital offers itself as the signifier of a desiring self, the hysteric erases it, eradicating the genital from psychic vision, replacing it with the smooth surface of the sexless torso.

Freud made the genital the sign of sexual difference and designated the boy's penis as an object of female envy, a highly complex argument that has been oversimplified, but has also unfortunately diverted attention away from other aspects of the child's struggle to identify with the genital. We might say that sexuality now presents the child with the psychic task of both meeting and fulfilling the challenge of the genital.

Consider the penis.

Out front, so to speak, it signifies excitement whether the self wishes it to or not. Erections point something out, but is the self up to the act suggested by the shape? Who leads whom? A physical object with psychic correlates, it eventually signifies penetration of x, initially standing for the vagina, which comes to signify any object to be penetrated. But as the first object is the vagina, what that object itself stands for assumes critical significance for the psychology of exploration.

Does the penis signify procreation? For Ferenczi ([1923] 1938), it was that object through which men and women fulfilled a phylogenetic wish to return to the lost sea from which the race emerged. As the uterus was that lost sea, does the penis in intercourse represent urgent longing in men and women to return to their origins?

The castration complex proper, however, focuses on the child's use of fantasy to fill the gap created by the absent penis, embodied for the child in the girl's anatomy. Where is it? What has happened to it? And who did it? These become seminal questions posed by each gender's specific place in this order of anxiety. From these questions spring – at least in the psychoanalyst's imagination – a remarkable number of theories, but I shall limit myself to only a few that bear on our topic. As these questions about the genitalia arrive as part and parcel of the sexual epiphany described above, the one who is supposed to know the answer to them – unsurprisingly enough – is the one who is presumed to have disposed of the phallus: none other than the father. Indeed, it may well be that this is the point in the archaic imaginary when God the mother is usurped by God the father, as now the penis-as-organ is supplanted by the phallus as signifier of all penetration into the world of mothers and babies.

The mother now becomes a sphinx whose silence accompanies a catastrophe that can only be remedied by solving her riddle through thought and speech. But the child's sexual epiphany is projected back into her. There is something learned here which cannot be spoken for. There is something lost here which cannot be remembered. At the moment of entering the family and the social order as a fully speaking participant the child's relation to the mother is silenced by discovery of sexuality, posing questions beyond any immediate answering. Even if childhood and adolescence constitute a psycho-biological answering of this question, the child inscribes in his or her memory the experience of trauma built around the epiphany: a realisation that leaves the infant–mother relation mute. In analysis this mute love relation, operating in and through silence, is an intrinsic part of the erotic transference of the hysteric, who insists that his or her love of the analyst not be spoken. Even as the analyst requests in one way or the other that it be spoken, the patient cathects the couch, the silence, the corpuscular ambience (two bodies breathing together) and erotises the transference, which becomes the love object. This demand – that the patient's love survives the analyst's interpretations and even the patient's reports – is based on the structure of each individual's erotic attachment to the mother.

An image.

A small child is sitting on mother's lap, whilst she talks to a friend. The child puts his hand on the mother's mouth. She loses verbal coherence. What emerges is a mumble. A mother mumble. The child is delighted. But if the mother tries to remove the hand, or tries to speak in spite of it, the child and mother enter into a more determined combat.

Why does the child try to silence the mother's speech? Is it to preserve her in the pre-symbolic order? Is she meant to be the sphinx who will not tell? In silencing with the hand, it joins the mouth in a bond between two bodies, first smashed upon the lips, then vigorously trying to get inside her mouth. But the mother insists upon speaking.

Does she betray the child when she tells what has been said and done? Is this the betrayal of contents? This is difficult to see, because very often what she speaks of are the child's accomplishments. Instead, it is a betrayal of form. She is not meant to report on their universe. Words themselves betray.

Children must now think themselves again. Certain immediate preoccupations – such as figuring out gender – are forms of recuperation from the disturbing change of the object world.

Psychoanalytical theories of the castration complex may, ironically, mirror the child's own fantasies, as there are a remarkable number of imaginings about who has the phallus and what it means. But all analysts who adhere to this theory would agree that in the child's imaginary the father becomes a fearsome figure who threatens the self with mutilation; and in the child's movement into the oedipal stage efforts to resolve the desire for the mother will be saturated and compromised by anxiety in relation to the father, who bars the relation to the mother with imagined deep threats. As argued earlier, the father's violence is energised by the child's repudiation (castration) of sexuality and re-energised by its continuous emergence and denial.

If the boy's penis is out there as an appendage apparently privileging its possessor, the vagina seems to raise questions. It is not visible to its bearer. Indeed, a girl can choose not to examine it for as long as she wishes. As a psychic correlate, it signifies that object of desire which remains hidden until such time as the bearer seeks to explore it. If the boy is continuously familiar with his penis, the girl is not so familiar with her vagina and as such it is more likely to be elaborated through the imaginary. Later, when she takes up a mirror and spreads her legs to begin exploration, she will have to part its subtle folds and upon doing so will discover a multi-layered object that opens and reopens. The self looks inside its body. Quite profound questions arise about whether the girl wishes to explore x (any potential opening) that sponsors derived questions such as whether one would or would not wish to look further into the matters of life. Usually, it is in adolescence that young women feel more inclined to examine more completely the vagina. If so, then they will customarily be parting the pubic hair, opening up the labia, and by getting the self in the right light, finding the clitoris and searching into the interiors of the vagina. Upon inspection, the young woman faces an interesting juxtaposition of the imaginary and the real object. For some, the object emerging out of the real seems oddly different from the imaginary vagina and it may sponsor a kind of dread.

Some women feel the vagina is a disturbing orifice that leaks dead babies and 'yucky' substances, and admits unpleasant penetrating objects such as the penis. Other women grow up feeling that the vagina is the birthplace of the world. Both of these views tend to be the thinking of the child, whilst a woman who has matured will come to understand her vagina as an 'object' with complex associations and deep personal meanings.

Boys and girls of 3 are psychically bisexual. They possess the opposite genital in the imaginary. Setting aside the fact that both are envious of the genitalia of the parents, the girl's preoccupation with the penis is more likely to be envy of the genital that can easily be seen, but, ironically, as her own genital will be left up to her imagination for some time, she begins weaving stories about the genitalia and their significance long before the male does.

But as the genitalia are the agents of sexuality, the hysteric's solution is to 'disavow' them, in order to ascend to a 'higher' level of function. As such, basic psychic functions deriving out of acceptance of the genitalia – the penetrating search for answers, the opening-up of areas of investigation – are suspended. Instead, the hysteric cultivates a type of ignorance that becomes crucial to sustaining the little-boy or little-girl self.

Adult hysterics are tempted to abandon sexuality because it is 'too complicated'. One patient ended all her sexual encounters with men or women after several months: 'Sexuality makes things too complicated between us.' Her last partner rejected her as childish and sexually immature. She knew this to be true and frankly asserted that she did not want to have a sexual relation, arguing that if her partner really loved her then sex should not come between them. This opposition between love and sexuality is a core feature of hysteria, which only makes sense if we see that the hysteric views sexuality as a form of separation from maternal-like love.

As children they will often indicate the future of sexual renunciation by siding with the vulnerable aspects of the self, negating more adaptive parts of the personality. They may refuse social activities or stay home from school in order to receive maternal care. They may become sickly and require nursing care from the mother or her surrogate. Presenting the body as an object that requires nursing signifies demand of a nursing other who also sees the body as afflicted and in need of continuous restoration.

Entering the oedipal period, the child is also confused about how to come to terms with parental sexuality and one's place in the family. The natural tendency is to see the father as a sexually inappropriate villain who has intruded upon the child's relation to the mother; but as the mother chooses him, and as sexuality must be negated in order to be psychologically born again as a boy or a girl, Jesus to the mother's Mary, the hysteric may accept a desexualised father and mother to go along with the desexualised self.

Psychoanalysis offers many differing theories of psychic complexities imagined to be particular to each gender. Whilst there are certainly differing psychic challenges to each gender in its affiliation with each parent, it is not possible to construct a theory of hysteria – or any other character, for that matter – around sexual difference as such. As will become apparent in the following chapters, I do not think hysteria is a complex particular to women; indeed, I think there are as many male as there are female hysterics. (Male impotence, for example, is a common conversion symptom in men, as are headaches, bad backs, and the like.) Genders may come equipped with preordained psychic maps; but the sexuality that psychoanalysis addresses is the self's psychic position *in* the sexual: either in fantasy, in enactment or in object relations. A heterosexual man's unconscious sexual fantasies could be lesbian; a homosexual woman's sexual fantasies could be heterosexual. How people conceive of themselves consciously is of course important to anyone's right of self declaration, but it does not necessarily equate to the psychoanalyst's interpretation of what constitutes sexuality.I do not think the female and the male hysteric divide over the core complex of hysteria itself. Each gender experiences its sexuality as disruptive and seeks desexualisation as the solution. Nor do I think the sexual classes – heterosexual or homosexual – divide over the complex of the hysteric. Both homosexuals and heterosexuals may be hysteric, each sharing the self's opposition to the disruptive effects of the drive. Each class would find its own path to transcendence and each would share all the other traits of the hysteric.

It is more than ironic that the hysteric, the character who privileges sexuality as the divisive issue of a lifetime, does not turn his or her identity on the lathe of sexual difference. Indeed, the very drive to oblate the genitals and cover them over with a sexless genital eradicates the significance of gender-in-itself. All that remains for any hysteric is what remains for the normal person: that being a girl or a boy involves the self in a set of desires and identifications on offer in the course of the self's development in family life.

The most prominent paradox of the hysteric, however, is the exchange of carnal sexuality – specifically, the genital drive – for spiritual sexuality. Where once the body and its drives prevailed upon the self to accept the animal within, the hysteric vigorously refuses this logic, but uncannily inverts carnal excitation into spiritual excitation. In 'Petrarchan love', the self is afflicted by the sight of the love object. The self cannot touch this other, but this seeming frustration is transformed into an extraordinary teasing, which endlessly drives the self to repeated imaginings of the love object, which in turn is cumulatively removed to even higher ground. The self's carnal body is contrasted with its other body, its soul, which will touch its love object through the purity of love itself. Any suggestion otherwise, especially the notion that the self might give in to its body cravings, would destroy the soul's right to its love object.

The hysteric's sexuality, then, is not simply based on sacrifice of the body; it can be achieved only if the body is eradicated from consideration. Yet how can we square this with the fact that hysterics do make love?

As we shall see in subsequent chapters, this is no simple matter; but, to prevent confusion, it is important to clarify now that any hysteric in love is inside an auto-suggestive spell. Under the pressure of the instinct and/or the sexual demand of the other, they may enter the sex space and make love, but they mentally eradicate this carnal engagement, and in its place put the soul. This is hysterical bliss. As the body generates its excitation the hysteric is frenzied by his or her own redirection of the instinct, routing it upward toward higher and purer forms of passion, from where it is now blessed and then returned to the body for its newly directed sexual–spiritual engagement with the other. Sacrificial pain becomes the passion.

Sexual excitation is transformed into spiritual excitation. But this transformation is always, at least unconsciously, linked to the psychic, if not real, impossibility of the self's intercourse with the other. The hysteric's solution is rather ingenious, shoving the dilemma into the mainstream topoi of Western letters: out of unrequited love the self discovers the power of higher forms.

Sir Thomas Wyatt's 'Description of the contrarious passions in a lover' begins:

> I find no peace, and all my war is done;
> I fear and hope; I burn, and freeze like ice;

It ends:

> I love another, and thus I hate myself;
> I feed me in sorrow, and laugh in all my pain.
> Likewise displeaseth me both death and life,
> And my delight is causer of this strife.

Unrequited love, perhaps ordained by chance, is the path selected by the hysteric, who would agree with Wyatt that it is a hot and cold passion and that this kind of love necessitates a hatred of the body self, where in self affliction one finds a bliss that seems to be the way one can touch the other. Whilst masochism in the pervert remembers excitation from the real (see Chapter 14), the hysteric's masochism is the transformation of body excitation from its carnal logic to an erotic undoing, from the pulsions moving toward its orgasm to the waves of despair created by the self's abstention from sexual life with the other.

Note

1 *Guardian*, 14 July 1997, G2, p. 7.

Chapter 3

Sexuality and its transformations

Loss of innocence imposed by the body is shocking enough to sponsor a violent unconscious refusal of the body. Few of Freud's cases reveal this trauma as clearly as 'Dora', the story of an 18-year-old girl. Distressed by the sexual advances of a middle-aged family friend, Herr K, she reports him to her father, who refers her to Freud.

At one point, Freud considers an episode when she found Herr K's attempt to kiss her only repelling. 'She summoned up an infantile affection for her father,' he wrote, 'so that it might protect her against her present affection for a stranger' (1905a: 86). Yet if her affection for Herr K motivated this summoning, her repulsion also expresses the more traumatic effect of her awareness of paternal (and maternal) sexuality. At the least, she was also fleeing from her sexual father, and it was the effort to reassert a desexualised self that motivated much of her anguish.

Indeed, Freud speculates that Dora's father, who had syphilis in his youth, infected both the mother and Dora herself, a fact that Dora discovered when overhearing an account of her father's sexual history, so in this sense the father's sexuality pollutes the child's and the mother's pre-sexual innocence.

Dora's dream life reflects this core trauma. The first dream is described as follows (1905a: 64):

> A house was on fire. My father was standing beside my bed and woke me up. I dressed quickly. Mother wanted to stop and save her jewel case; but Father said: 'I refuse to let myself and my two children be burnt for the sake of your jewel case.' We hurried downstairs, and as soon as I was outside I woke up.

Freud sees this dream as a disguised expression of Dora's guilt over her masturbations, which excited her in the night to the point of bed-wetting. Jewel case, 'Schmuckkästchen', is a 'term commonly used to describe female genitals that are immaculate and intact' (p. 91). The jewel case, according to Freud, signifies sexual temptations, as Herr K had given Dora a jewel case, which also represents a masturbatory object. For Freud, the father's comment disguises his reproach to the masturbating child, who will consume the house with her passion.

That seems to me only half the story, at the least, for it marginalises Dora's shock over sexuality and her effort to reassert her mother's virginity. The mother's wish to save her jewel case – in the scene of sexual passion – may be a projection of the child's wish that the mother preserve her virginity in the face of the contaminating effects of sexuality, a sexuality that brings disease and madness into the safety of the home.

Dora's conflict becomes clearer in a second dream. Wandering through strange streets, she discovers her home; she enters, whereupon she finds a note from her mother declaring that as Dora had left the house without parental knowledge, the mother had not sent her a note informing her of her father's death. Now that he was dead she could return. Dora proceeds to a railway station, sees herself in a thick wood, meets a man who offers to accompany her, declines his suggestion, finds the station, reaches her home, and hears from a servant that her mother is at the cemetery. Freud presses Dora to recall where she was wandering in the dream and she remembers declining the company of a male cousin upon a visit to a Dresden art gallery, as she preferred to go alone. 'She remained two hours in front of the Sistine Madonna, rapt in silent admiration. When I asked her what had pleased her so much about the picture she could find no clear answer to make. At last she said: "The Madonna"' (p. 96).Freud regards her association as an identification with a young man's wandering and later adds that the dream contains a fantasy of defloration, which raises anxiety that is dealt with by evoking the image of the Sistine Madonna. Freud gets very close indeed to grasping the function of the pure virgin, but stops short of suggesting that the appearance of sexuality in the first place (the male cousin who wishes to accompany her; the man who offers to take her to the station) evokes the wish to return to the Madonna mother. With the death of the father, the daughter is allowed by the mother to return home. This father – who embodies sexuality – must be killed if the child is to return to immaculate maternal care.

Freud rightly emphasises Dora's sexual jealousy of her mother, yet her disappointment with her father for preferring other women also testifies to her passionate participation in family life. Her conflict reflects the return of the child to family life after the urge to seek refuge in the Madonna mother. Freud saw only her denial of her wishes, not the reason for a primary denial of sexuality itself. In this respect, he also failed to see that in addressing the desires of the 18-year-old girl without understanding how she experienced sexuality in the first place (including Freud's matter-of-fact discussion of it), he ignored the child who insisted upon standing rapt before the Madonna. She lapsed into silence when he asked after the Madonna, affirming in silence her love of the pre-verbal mother. As if to sanctify this return, she was to give Freud just two more hours of her presence before leaving analysis, something which did not escape his attention.

Looking at the Madonna, Dora would have directed her gaze up to the mother's face. In Christian theology, especially in the medieval cosmologies, the upper part of the body suggests transcendence, as one looks *up* towards the deity. This is the food of Christian love, and it is based on the infant's dwelling in the eyes of the mother, who provides her milk and her love. It will be some time before something happens from below that creates a new order of things, disrupting the heavenly gaze. The Christian world assigns this rupture to the Devil, who embodies all that disturbs the sacred order. As Dora exemplified, and as Freud failed to see – so taken up was he in advocating the universality of human sexuality – sexual urges seem to destroy the self's relation to the sacred primary object, unless they can be transported from carnality to spirituality, with the soul as a stand-in for the genital.

Later on, Freud would concentrate on another recognition. He saw in the young child's denial of sexual difference the basis of psychosis, indicating a refusal of reality that would have repercussions later. Today, analysts would argue that this refusal is the formation of hysterical psychosis, as the schizophrenias, for example, involve an oblation of the mental apparatus that could perceive an unwanted reality from a very early stage of life. Indeed, much of Bion's work, for example, is concerned with attacks on linking driven by the psychotic part of the person-ality's refusal to allow unwanted connections of thought to be made. There is an equivalent form of attack on linking with the hysteric, only here the severance of a link is to sexual mental contents, evoked in the self or proposed by the other. A violent form of innocence is instituted, to negatively hallucinate sexual representations in the world and to repress them when they emerge from the instincts.

Given the complexity of human psychic development, it is no wonder that Freud reminded his readers that all persons suffer an hysterical stage and that the so-called 'normal' person is only more normal – more normal by degrees rather than by quality. Nevertheless, it is useful to have a concept of the normal child.

Another of Freud's cases, 4-year-old Little Hans, is awakened by sexual excitement into lusting after several neighbours, and after just about any little girl he comes across. And real life offers real sex objects, such as a mother and father in bed. 'Lying in bed with his father or mother was a source of erotic feelings in Hans just as it is in every other child' (1905a: 17) and Hans creates a special word – 'coax', which means to caress – repeatedly to call his mother to physical intimacy. It is worth pointing out that the 'source' of this excitation is not simply instinctual, as it derives from the physical presence of the parents' bodies. This helps us understand why children more or less determine their sexual orientation. They choose sex objects because the intensity of their sexual urges demands this, so an other will be selected for the romantic elaboration – and thus diminution – of sexual states of mind. Object love at this stage complies with the child's need to satisfy his or her drives; and the availability of the other as the object through which these drives may be satisfied is immediately apparent to the child, who finds through the other what Freud calls the 'erotic sense' (1905a: 17).

A famous idea of Bion's is that a thought requires a thinker; the mind evolves in order to think thoughts arising. Freud's theory is that instincts require an object; object relations derive from the instincts arising.

Hans tells his parents that he would like to sleep with Mariedl, an older girl. Freud speculates that 'there can be no doubt that lying beside [his parents] had aroused erotic feelings in him; so that his wish to sleep with Mariedl had an erotic sense as well' (1905a: 17). The feelings arriving out of experience contribute to an increased 'sense', which in turn demands an object. It is Hans's discovery of the other through whom the sense can be satisfied – his mother and other females – that contributes to the positive (i.e. normal) side of the solution to his dilemma. The hysterical strategy would be to effect the opposite: to find some way to deny to the other those erotic states that are driving the self toward sexual bliss between two beings.

In many of Freud's writings which followed, the child's gender identifications and choices of sex object are understood to be a resolution of castration anxieties. But Freud's instruction to Little Hans's father is very interesting and suggests an earlier reason. 'The truth was, his father was to say, that he was very fond of his mother and wanted to be taken into her bed. The reason he was afraid of horses now was that he had taken so much interest in their widdlers. He himself had noticed that it was not right to be so very much preoccupied with widdlers, even with his own, and he was quite right in thinking this' (1905a: 28). Note that Freud does not say that it is not right for the boy to think of sleeping with his mother. Indeed, both the father and Freud more or less accept that the mother will take Hans to her bed for 'coaxing'. It is masturbation that he is ordered to abandon by the mother, the father and the doctor.

On 2 March, when Hans shows renewed fear of horses, his father says that this 'nonsense' is due to his lack of 'walks', but Hans quickly replies, 'Oh no, it's so bad because I still put my hand to my widdler every night' (p. 30). Freud muses: 'Doctor and patient, father and son, were therefore at one in ascribing the chief share in the pathogenesis of Hans's present condition to his habit of masturbating' (p. 30), although he concludes the sentence by adding that there were other 'significant factors'. Indeed, Hans's desire for his mother, his fear of his father and the well-known themes of the oedipal conflict are all significant, though they derive from the abandonment of auto-erotism.

Furthermore, this abandonment will be accomplished by directing the erotic sense toward sex objects – mothers, other girls, etc. – at the same time that the energy behind erotic self-stimulation is discouraged. The struggle is between the narcissistic envelope of the auto-erotic, in which the child can conjure any object of desire in his or her own mind, a strategy which would certainly not propagate the race, and the allo-erotic. Parents seduce children away from the auto-erotic, as if Echo finally lured Narcissus away from the love of his own reflection. At the same time, by discouraging auto-erotic stimulation, parents diminish this source of excitation at the very point of having secured a transfer of the object of desire, from self to other.

As previously discussed, this fortuitously dovetails with the arrival of the mother as a sex object, which excitation, ironically enough, the child will seek to discharge through masturbation, enveloping the other in the circuits of auto-erotism. However, this effort to bring the mother back into one's own body, through the genital object, is defeated by parental admonitions about self-stimulation, accompanied by transformed parental seduction of the child: now the parents elicit the child's desire for their desire, to have the child exchange acute love of their bodies for love of their love and guidance.

The situation is compounded by the function of the auto-erotic in children. For it is around 15 months that children begin to masturbate, although prior to this they will have received countless maternal caresses of their body. As we shall argue in the next chapter, the mother's desire of the self's infantile body is crucial to one's sexual well-being, but if we regard the first stages of genital masturbation as a moment when deferred infantile sexuality (as in a *Nachträglichkeit*) is now 'remembered', then the self-stimulating 15-month-old will simultaneously recall to his or her bodily pleasures the mother's hands. If the mother has understimulated the infant then auto-erotism will stand in for the lack of maternal sensorial care (Heimann, personal communication in 1976), but if the mother was deeply seductive, then the child will make the unconscious link between self-stimulation and maternal love. This is the ready-made ground, as it were, for the sexual epiphany of the 3-year-old, which will be yet another remembering of the mother–infant love relation.

The psycho-logic of the scene of the 3-year-old is uncanny. The child experiences an increase in genital sensations in relation to the mother, but it is fundamentally a self-stimulated object love that naturally evokes prior proto-incests. Self-stimulation regulates the excitement, returning the child to his or her own body – thus modifying incestuous object love – but parental intervention requires the child to give it up, although it now serves to discharge the self of excitation aroused by the mother's body. The child's solution is therefore refused, as if saying: 'I think the solution to this dilemma is that I masturbate and you masturbate me', and as if the parent replied: 'No, you must give that up.' What is a child to do with this refusal of the perceived solution? At this point erotisation is exchanged for identification, or, more exactly, identification is erotised. The child is given a set of 'proper' habits, which, in many respects, are reaction formations to the child's own infantile sexuality. The libido, formerly directed to the expression of these traits, now finds gratification in opposition to them, whilst this in turn earns parental love.

The child identifies with the mother or with the father, desiring a sex object in line with the norm; this is now more easily secured, as the child is already in a sexual latency of sorts when coming to this decision. What has been castrated is not the penis that would direct itself towards the mother's body, but quite the opposite: the penis or the clitoris that gives the self its own pleasure has been subdued. When Hans's mother sees him touching his penis at 3½ she says: 'If you do that, I shall send for Dr A to cut off your widdler. And then what'll you widdle with?' (1905a: 7, 8). The struggle throughout his early treatment is to get the child to give up masturbation and, if anything, to take the mother – and others – as proper sex objects, to be sexually possessed in the future.

The child's sexual epiphany involves a curious disturbance of the self's excitations. The self's own body is quite capable of giving it all that it sexually desires at this point. Masturbation is frowned upon, however, because there is something in the narcissism of auto-erotism that cuts the self off from the other; if practised to the exclusion of allo-erotic investment, ultimately it would threaten the survival of the race. The child having been urged by the parents to give up the body as the source of sexual excitement, the father becomes the law-maker of this abandonment in the child's psychic reality, presiding over a castration that eliminates the child's sexual means. This relinquishment leads to an immediate diminution of sexual excitation, and the child is invited to slot into the world of selves and others in a somewhat less sexually possessed frame of mind.

In his discussion of Little Hans Freud says that 'we may assume' that, since the boy had been in 'a state of intensified sexual excitement, the object of which was his mother', 'he found an incidental channel of discharge for it by masturbating every evening and in that way obtaining gratification' (1905a: 119). By giving up masturbation, the child is encouraged to give up an important means of gratification in relation to the mother, albeit one that involves the self living separately from the object of desire. However, if we understand this abandonment as the mid-point in a sexual realisation – from the original increase in genital excitation and its attachment to objects of desire, to the recognition of the differences between the sexes and the fears of genital mutilation – then the dictate that self-stimulation must be suppressed is a form of proactive castration, as the child's sex life has been 'gently' attacked by the parents.

To put it differently, parents organise a seduction by the mother, moving the child from the autistic sexuality of the auto-erotic to desire for the mother and her sex object, the father. 'But this must stop' is an injunction against self-stimulation: 'You may have me later' is the promise of deferral. Indeed, all along mother and father propose themselves as sex objects to the child, seducing the boy into object love of the mother and the girl into object love of the father, marrying the object of the instinct (an auto-erotic object) to the other of sexual fulfilment. When the marriage is complete, the child 'realises' his or her sexuality as passion for the sex object as other.

As early as 1893, in 'On the psychical mechanism of hysterical phenomena', Freud notes the work of parental seduction:

> The child takes both of its parents, and more particularly one of them, as the object of its erotic wishes. In so doing, it usually follows some indication from its parents whose affection bears the clearest characterisation of a sexual activity, even though of one that is clearly inhibited in its aim.
>
> (p. 47)

Later on, in the 'Three Essays' (1905b), having said that the mother 'clearly treats [the infant] as a substitute for a complete sexual object', Freud concludes that by 'rousing her child's sexual instinct and preparing for its later intensity' she is 'only fulfilling her task in teaching the child to love' (p. 223) – to which Winnicott would later add that the infant believes this erotic moment to be his or her human right and the breast the mother of invention.

Freud refers to paternal seduction in 'A child is being beaten' (1919), when he writes that 'the affections of the little girl are fixed on her father, who has probably *done all he could to win her love*, and in this way has sown the seeds of an attitude of hatred and rivalry towards her mother' (p. 10, my italics).

The mother and father seduce the infantile instinct. They want themselves to be taken as its object. The instinct – if we allow its theoretical existence as a primal fantasy – drives toward the breast like a lover saturated with pre-existent erotic knowledge.

The parents having successfully seduced the child into desire of the other, new anxieties arise in the child – especially those of genital mutilation – and fulfilment is deferred. In the ensuing latency, however, children turn to their natural sex objects, most easily other children, to bring sexual states of excitation in relation to the body of the other.

We might think of this exchange, then, as an ordinary hysteria on the part of the parents and of culture, one that insists upon a temporary desexualisation of the self. Freud makes it clear in his account of the treatment of Dora that her symptoms partly derived from the effects of childhood masturbation, from which he draws a link to hysteria proper. 'Hysterical symptoms hardly every appear so long as children are masturbating', he writes, 'but only afterwards, when a period of abstinence has set in; they form a substitute for masturbatory satisfaction, the desire for which continues to persist in the unconscious until another and more normal kind of satisfaction appears' (1905a: 25). And what might that normal satisfaction be? That would depend on 'the possibility of a hysteria being cured by marriage and normal sexual intercourse' (p. 79). How so, we might ask? In effect, this child's family – and we can include Freud as an extended member – collaborates in an hysterical response to the child's emergent sexuality, when they demand he or she give up his genital excitations. If this intensifies the child's romantic love for the mother – as it would seem to do with both Hans and Dora – this is the ordinary outcome of sexual abstinence and the subsequent pining for a love object, a form of suffering which Freud – who put off his marriage for some years – would well have understood. But the family's intervention necessitates a deferral of the child's sexuality, not, we might add, because the family fears that children will seek *actual* love with the objects of desire (in the numerous accounts of the child's heartfelt expression of passion, the parents and Freud virtually bask in the sweetness of the claims), but because the family recognises in self-stimulation a route the self could take that would break up the family structure under the force of separate instincts, finding sufficient fulfilment through internal objects without the need for actual others.

'Investigation of the childhood history of hysterical patients', writes Freud in 'Some general remarks on hysterical attacks', 'shows that the hysterical attack is designed to take the place of an *auto-erotic* satisfaction previously practised and since given up' (1909a: 232). Indeed, the 'loss of consciousness' typical of the hysterical attack is 'derived from the fleeting but unmistakable lapse of conscious-ness which is observable at the climax of every intense sexual satisfaction, including auto-erotic ones' (p. 233). Hysteria, then, carries forward the secret life of the self's auto-erotism.

In 'Hysterical phantasies and their relation to bisexuality' (1908) Freud links auto-erotic moments to the ordinary daydream, which is simply a vector of the auto-erotic in ordinary life. He draws attention to a daydreamer walking along the street, so self-absorbed that as he approaches the end of his fantasy his steps quicken marking 'the climax of the imagined situation' (p. 160). Hysterical attacks are nothing more, he argues, than 'an involuntary irruption of day-dreams of this kind' (p. 160), although they are based on unconscious fantasies which, Freud claims, are 'identical with the phantasy which served to give him sexual satisfaction during a period of masturbation' (p. 161).

It is interesting to note Freud's effort to include the many dimensions of the castration complex in his 1924 essay 'The Dissolution of the Oedipus Complex'. Squarely facing the fact that the child's masturbations elicit threats of castration from the parents – especially the mother – Freud writes that 'what brings about the destruction of the child's phallic genital organisation is this threat of castration' (p. 175). But not immediately, because the boy does not believe in the threat. It is only sometime later, when 'a *fresh* experience comes his way, that the child begins to reckon with the possibility of being castrated' (p. 175); that new experience is the sight of the female genitals. 'With this, the loss of the penis becomes imaginable, and the threat of castration takes its deferred effect' (p. 176). The auto-erotic passions become 'only a genital discharge of the sexual excitation belonging to the complex' Freud argues. This scenario is the one imagined for the boy. What of the girl? 'At this point our material – for some incomprehensible reason – becomes far more obscure and full of gaps', writes Freud (p. 177), leaving us to wonder whether he was conscious or not of what is meant by 'full of gaps'. For, certainly, the site of the supposed castration is a gap, a gap which sight of the penis – or the fetish – is meant to fill.

In this same essay Freud considered the other forms of castration, such as weaning and giving up faeces, but he claims there is no evidence to suggest that with the threat of castration these precursive or little castrations have any effect. That must await sight of the female genital.

What if that sight, however, is exactly as he says: the signifier 'full of gaps'. A signifier that indicates a plurality of gaps. Read this way, sight of the genital becomes, for interesting reasons, a vision of that which takes away. And if so, does this sight become meaningful only when the boy links it to the removal of his penis, or is it a wish that the castration one must fear is the loss of the penis in an imaginary intercourse with the mother? Would the creation of this myth fill in many gaps, left in mind, were they not filled up with this particular theory at this particular moment?

I do not quarrel with Freud's insistence that genital difference deeply affects psychic structure, nor do I think he is wrong to specify sight of the vagina as particularly troubling to small children. I think, however, that he has characteristically rushed in with the genital too early, wishing away even more disturbing psychic elements, like a boy at swordplay. The mystery that Freud supposes woman to be, conjured by him on innumerable occasions when he tries to find a place for her in his otherwise phallocentric theory, is the presence of the overdetermined gap that cannot be filled by a single idea . . . or object. This gap, out of which all of us are born and to which we return, this opening from which the self emerges into human existence, to be subsequently returned to the inorganic – realisation of this place is a most impressive discovery indeed.

For Freud it signifies the place where one's imagination loses the self's penis. In fact, the penis – representative of the self – has already lost its place. The self has already been removed, not simply in the prior removals – from breast, faeces, etc. – but from a world which later will be retrospectively idealised: a world of innocence, a world of dependence on a loving mother, before realisation of sexuality ejected it from Eden. Sight of the vagina is akin to mental sight, to seeing for the first time where one is, and what one has lost. Of course, one discovers parental sexuality in a new way, but one is also confronted by the mystery of woman, or more correctly, woman as bearer of the mysteries, especially those known by the pre-verbal sphinx mother, silenced by language.

We cannot accept Freud's truncation of the function of the auto-erotic, now put entirely at the disposal of the oedipal complex, although no doubt it does serve to discharge the self of excitations operating in relation to the parent's body. But, in that respect, self-stimulation has served as the engine of excitation and its discharge, from the beginning of life. Ordinarily the mother has always offered her body – as an alternative to the infant's own body – as the vehicle for stimulation and discharge. Parents threaten castration in order to move the child toward his or her future sex objects: 'Stop playing with yourself and start imagining life as an adult.'

Typical of his own way of revising his simplifications, Freud corrected his 1924 paper a year later with 'Some psychical consequences of the anatomical distinction between the sexes' (1925). His wording evokes even more powerful senses of the parental aim to end the child's masturbations: 'the masturbation of early childhood, the more or less *violent suppression* of which by those in charge of the child sets the castration complex in action' (my italitcs). And then, repeating his statement of the previous year that 'this masturbation is attached to the Oedipus complex', Freud concludes that there is a 'second possibility' that 'is by far the more probable'. And what is that? It is that 'masturbation . . . makes its first appearance spontaneously as an activity of a bodily organ and is only brought into relation with the Oedipus complex at some later date' (p. 250). Brought in, that is, by parental seduction of the child's heterosexual desire (or homosexual desire, if the case so be), lest the child remain in the autistic universe of imagined objects and hand-held reliefs. 'Object-choice pushes auto-erotism into the background' wrote Freud in 1893 (p. 45).

The child must be seduced into his or her future. A future which, within the child's present, functions as a carrier of what is being deferred. The deferring of sexual realisation into the future saturates the self's inner sense of the future as libidinally promising. It is this imaginary relation to his or her future that the hysteric partly refuses.

Hysterical symptoms not only ensure the private continuation of auto-erotic life, they also constitute a rebellion against the claims of object love. They nurture – indeed, *drive* – the idiom of thought that we know as daydreaming, but which Freud unmistakably sees as an extension of auto-erotism into ordinary life: the street walker, Freud notes, is cut off from fellow walkers, absorbed in the auto-erotic universe of privately imagined gratifications.

Unconscious fantasy is a compromise between the purely auto-erotic and the allo-erotic, as the self stimulates its body (pure auto-erotism), but entertains a fantasy of the other (allo-erotic). In normal development the self gives up the priority of the auto-erotic and finds in the other a solution to the agonies of a repudiated sexuality; but, according to Freud, the hysteric will seek a compromise by abandoning auto-erotism, to find an alternative in the symptom, a stand-in for auto-erotic life: 'in this way the giving up of the habit of masturbation is in fact undone' (1908:162).

The non-hysteric, as suggested, has exchanged the auto-erotic for the future and is already practising it by identification in the fields of play. The energy for normal development resides in the promise of sexual gratification, deferred now to fulfil all later. The child is savvy enough to say: 'One day I will marry x.' This exchange – 'You must give up the auto-erotic and one day we will give you x' – accomplishes the transformation from excitement to identification, from the pulsions of the present to desire which operates through the future. Desire accepts a deferral and when the self falls in love, it is a marriage in the present of the past's future: 'Ah, I knew this would come true. Here you are!'

Thinking futuristically, then, is an erotic drive, receiving the libido that would have circled through auto-erotism around memories of past bliss (the breast recalled in thumb-sucking) and transferring it to the future, in the self's dream of an ideal sex object waiting in the wings of reality. The love objects of the past and of the future are both constructed in the self's fantasy life, but the memorial sex object would always be enough and the self would never need to negotiate with reality, whereas the future sex object must be vigorously sought in the outside world. Psycho-development is thus propelled by the sexual drive, and the death instinct – decathexis through immediately arranged for orgasm – is its opposite. Eros is reality oriented in spite of its nature; Thanatos hates the world of reality and uses fantasy to replace the real.

The child in the oedipal stage does not say 'I want to have intercourse with mummy' or 'I want to have intercourse with daddy', but 'I want to marry x'. The opposite-sex parent is seen as a rival who bars marriage in the present because of the superiority of the parent's genitals and the inferiority of the child's sexual capability. Once again, the self's body proves to be the problem. It is not the opposing parent alone, but rather the body which above all refuses the child's immediate romantic aspirations. This frustration with the body will be signified again and again by the hysteric.

By seducing the child into intense love of the mother, the human race uses her body as the lure to drive the child out of the solipsistic world of auto-erotism. At the point when this is accomplished – a moment that actually extends over some years – the father becomes an obstacle to both boy and girl, apparently to bar any further sexuality with the mother (partly true), but in fact the figure who bars infantile sexuality.

The Oedipus complex owes much to the phylogenetic investment on the part of the parents to seduce the child at that moment in his or her biological development when the child's genitality provides the mother as a sex object. The child is refused his or her solution to excitation – masturbation – which necessitates the search for a progressive sexual solution to the dilemma. He or she sexualises the future and, by identification, turns loss into sacrificial desire. Passion takes the place of abreactive self-stimulation. The parental prohibition against masturbation is not aimed against the child's sexuality, but against the infant's sex object (the genital alone) and towards the adult's sex object: the wonderful materialisation of the woman or man of one's dreams.

'Looking into the future' is an erotic particle, as the self envisions fulfilment of sexual promise. The future is resting on genital realisation, on the maturation of the self's sexuality; and as the oedipal child knows that he or she is genitally insufficient, the present is exchanged for the future, when the child will make real on the promise. This child of the Oedipus myth will return with the proper equipment to conquer the rival and copulate with the sex object.

When the future arrives – in adolescence – the child looks at the parent again and is blinded by what he or she sees. This is no longer a sex object. The future must again be deferred as the self tries to overcome the lost promise and the feeling of being betrayed by the early guarantees. Only now does the new sexual surge drive the adolescent to peer-group sex objects, and all seems promising in the real.

As the self moves into its future, then, it does so carrying lost erotic promises, biasing it to feel a certain betrayal. The Oedipus era was a moment of exchange. The child finds the mother to be a sex object that all along has been luring the infant out of auto-erotism. Both boy and girl lust after her body as the object of desire other than the self, a realisation that then drives the girl's love of the father, who embodies the pure otherness of desire. This exchange of narcissism for object love transforms sexual passion; sexual passion now drives romantic love, in which the immediate object of desire is sacrificed, thereby increasing its true value: deferral of gratification sexualises the future, which now promises a great reward in time. In this respect we may see how the economy of the auto-erotic is further cheated by the joint functions of sacrifice and deferral which comprise romantic love.

Deferral is required because if the race is to survive it cannot do so through generations of masturbators. The race must move itself from auto-erotic pleasure to allo-erotic desire, a transition it accomplishes through romantic love, which is based on sacrifice, deferral and sexual hope, all part of the foreplay of eventual sexual union.

The hysteric does not accept the above deferral and tries to sustain auto-erotic reveries based on an idealisation of the parents as asexual beings. The non-hysteric moves progressively into sexuality, the genitalia 'show up' the second time around – in adolescence – and there are sex objects available. But the hysteric is in grief because he or she has believed in the promise of virginal sexual realisations with the parent and the failure of this promise keeps the self in perpetual search for union of a non-sexual type with the ideal other: a mother or father *figure*.

One hysteric solution is to disavow the genitals and use the ecstasy of self-sacrifice to resurrect the virgin mother and her child lover. Another compromise is to co-opt the demand of reality by precocious – sometimes sexually adventurous – identifications, rushing through objects, seemingly deeply invested in the logic of the future, yet in truth using such precocity as a vehicle for a speedy return to the pre-adaptive world of infantile sexuality, supported by a parent who also declines the arrival of genitality. As the normal person courts the future, the hysteric lusts after the past.

When the hysteric marries it is to a heavily idealised figure, with intercourse often occurring as a kind of hypnotic moment – the genitalia obliterated from mind by the mesmerising effects of the sexual – or to a perpetually disappointing figure, with the ideal object carried in the mind in countless daydreams every day. Many couples in love return to a type of hysteria when the other becomes a deep ideal. This seems to be the promised fulfilment and the exchange is accepted. But the hysteric's love is deep auto-erotic preoccupation projected on to an other, and as soon as the other eventually differs from the internal one, there is bitter and confused disappointment. The non-hysteric finds in the compelling diversity of erotic knowledge a continuously new erotic other, which makes every intercourse different, and which delivers the self to a form of bliss unlike anything else in human life. The hysteric does not partake of erotic knowledge and makes love in either a blind or a detached manner, using the other as a figure with whom to masturbate. (As we shall discuss later, since erotic knowledge is based on the infant's love relation to the mother, the hysteric reproduces a body deprivation through the scarcity of erotic capability.)

Instead, the hysteric seeks in foreplay the endpoint of sexuality – a series of touchings which increase in excitation but which are never meant to find release in genital fulfilment, rather in withdrawal or frustration. Hysterical bliss thrives on this sacrifice, as self and other – brought to the point of sexual engagement – withdraw from it in order to testify to a greater or higher love. 'Wait. If you love me, you can wait.' In deferral is to be found true love. Sensing this conflict in the combat of love-making, the hysteric unconsciously arouses his or her body and the other in order to defeat the genital moment, each to turn away from that future into a past newly composed of memories of the erotic event, now a perfect collage of mnemic sensations ready for the self's auto-erotic reveries.

The auto-erotic denies the pleasures of the other. For Freud, this is at the heart of the hysteric's position. At the end of his brief essay 'Some general remarks on hysterical attacks' (1909a), Freud makes a stunning point. Hysterical 'loss of consciousness' is that kind of "*absence*" . . . derived from the fleeting but unmistakable lapse of consciousness which is observable at the climax of every intense sexual satisfaction, including auto-erotic ones' (p. 233). These 'absences' originate in early auto-erotic states of mind, when 'all the subject's attention is concentrated to begin with on the course of the process of satisfaction' and 'with the occurrence of the satisfaction, the whole of this cathexis of attention is suddenly removed, so that there ensues a momentary void in . . . consciousness'. From this, Freud makes the following link to a mental mechanism: 'This gap in consciousness, which might be termed a *physiological* one, is then widened in the service of repression, till it can swallow up everything that the repressing agency rejects' (p. 234).

Thus the hysteric finds ecstasy in a type of thinking: the orgasm of loss of consciousness. The mechanism of repression is not only sexualised, but becomes a form of auto-erotism, albeit exceedingly well disguised. This solution is rather remarkable. The hysteric transcends the contents of sexual life – thus achieving a type of purity – by identifying with that loss of consciousness occasioned by sexual ecstasy, which is 'widened in the service of repression', resulting in spells of erotic reveries with no contents. The sexuality is *in* this new loss and, ironically, elimination of the sexual contents becomes a new form of sexuality.[1]

Is it possible that as the self disappears from consciousness through the absences created by orgasm, it falls blissfully into the 'gap' from which it emerged? If knowledge of sexuality threatens the self's relation to the primary object, is repression then a skilful means of finding auto-hypnotic erotics at the moment of sexual exclusion? Is the wandering uterus of hysteria, which causes madness, the movement of that sea of which Ferenczi (1923) writes? Is there some phylogenetic knowledge playing itself out in this ancient theory of the wandering womb? If man (and woman) entered the gap and found that the womb had wandered off, would we then have no place to which we could return?

It is, as we shall see, no small part of the hysteric's sacrifice that he or she believes that sexuality divides the self from a mother that wanders off at the sight of sexual objects. 'What does a woman want?' bears a question to our species: 'What does sexuality expect from us?' A simple sensation? A penetration? For how far and how long? To what end? With what outcome? And can it be survived? The question that Freud assumed he could not answer on behalf of woman is the very question that woman is meant to bear for all of us: we do not know what she wants, we do not know what we want, we do not know what is wanted of us, and we are not sure – at any point in time – quite what we are 'getting ourselves into' through our furthered existence.

We shall return to these issues in subsequent chapters, but for now we ask ourselves another question: What predisposes children to hysteria? To put it another way, why do some undergo this rite of passage whilst others do not? To find an answer we must, as always, return to consider the origins of our being and the other who was there with us.

Note

1   The work of repression, therefore, is an auto-erotic action that gives to 'the absent' – contents or anorexias of character – the shape of desire. The act of splitting (and projective identifications) may 'carry' the erotic but in itself it bears the trace of oral and anal evacuation, not the ecstasy of the orgasmic. The reshaping of contents by splitting and projective identification reflects the 'earlier' in-formative communicatings of mother and infant, when early shapes of mental life are passed back and forth between the two, whilst the work of repression is inextricably derived from sexual life.

Chapter 4

In the beginning is the mother

When we mythologise the mother of the narcissist, we imagine a figure so frustrating that the infant eradicates his or her sense of the mother's otherness. Arnold Modell (1973) believes that she infuriates her infant to such an extent that the child deals with her unreliability by getting rid of dependence on the other, starting all over again with the self as stand-in for the other. When we think of the mother of the borderline, we imagine a figure who, for characterological or circumstantial reasons, is too sensorially and emotionally upsetting, and who unconsciously threatens the infant with her departure, encouraging her child to conjure turbulent states of mind because this is the body she offers. When we think of the mother of the schizophrenic, we consider that (again, for characterological or circumstantial reasons) the prospect of the infant perceiving her-in-herself is too endangering, to the point of threatening psychic annihilation, so the schizophrenic begins a radical process of abandoning his or her mental capabilities. If you do not have a mind sensitive to the nature of reality, then you are – so the strategy goes – less liable to experience pain brought about by the other.

Each of the above constructions is exceedingly one-sided: only the mother is imagined as disturbing, leaving the infant a kind of blank, seemingly derived from her failures. It is important to keep the limitations of these myths in mind, especially as it leaves out the infant's idiomatic distributions of love and hate. The borderline infant's turbulent frame of mind projects a chaotic object; the schizophrenic's psychic self-destruction creates an annihilating object; the narcissist's obtuseness fashions an out-of-touch primary object; and so the legend of the primary object could – if so wished – be constructed entirely out of projectile material.

As discussed in the Chapter 1, a great deal must be put in the name of the mother, in exactly the same way that fathers must bear unwanted parts of the child self, projected into his name. Parents know this. Small children blame the mother all the time for all kinds of things. And so too for the father. A large part of the skill of parenting is in accepting the projections, in the interests of the child's freedom of mind and expression, whilst at the same time allowing time and other frames of mind to enter the scene, so that these passing evacuations may be repaired by the child's sense of guilt and other frames of mind.

Parents accept vilification because being held responsible for the child's plight is partly accurate. The mother is meant to be the guardian of her infant's needs and when the child feels ill of mind or body, she may be held to blame. There is always a bad mother being held responsible for one's ills, just as there is a good mother responsible for one's well-being.

When we think of how a mother fails her infant we are forced to conclude that all infants are failed by the mother; indeed, childhood is a distressing time from which the self tries to recover over a lifetime.

When we think of how the mother fails the self, then, we are thinking of all that is subsumed under her name: the state and memories of being a foetus; the conditions of our birth; the primitive vicissitudes of the infant's feeble mental structure trying to process lived experience; and countless other frailties.

When thinking about the mother's name, we join the self in projection, putting all the ills of lived experience into 'mamma'. The primary object is constructed out of the infant's vision of the other, later to become an essential feature of the private dialogues within the self, when we take ourselves to be this other.

If the mother shall bear our distress with existence itself, she will perhaps be the associated beneficiary of our sense of aliveness. Essential to generative mothering is her erotic love of her infant, conveyed most particularly in the erotism of breast-feeding, which is a form of sexuality unto itself. With breast full, she often aches for the passionate attack of her hungry infant, whose suckling inspires a radiant pleasure that courses through her body. Maternal erotism would overwhelm the infant were it not for the power of the infant's instinct, as the drive ruthlessly to gratify hunger is a power arriving from within the infant, more than a match for the profound effect of maternal presence. The mother's pleasure in breast-feeding joins the infant's pleasure in feeding, registered through the mutuality of gaze that is as star-crossed as any lovers'. If the instinct creates its own mental object (the breast) and is driven by the urgent demand of the source (hunger), the erotic passion of the mother meets the infant's drive at the breast-feed – a crossroads not in Sophocles's *Oedipus Rex* – and both are transformed. The drive only seeks extinction of excitation, but it is forever altered by maternal erotism, which links the drive to the other's desire, out of which a new object is constructed. The new object is neither the object of the instinct (a purely mental representation) nor the object that is the mother as other: it is the object found by the intercourse between instinct and other. This is experience-become-object, laid down in psychic structure from the traces of mutual erotic experience.

Infant and mother are satiated by the breast-feed as a somatic, erotic and emotional experience. Fortunately, it is modified by quotidian factors: a mother may be too tired to enjoy it and is less than erotically inspired or inspiring, or she may be distracted, perhaps on the telephone talking to a friend. Likewise, the infant may not be in the mood for a feed, which instincts nonetheless force on him or her, causing the infant to approach the breast as if it were an annoying intrusion. These frequent alternatives to erotic passion infiltrate the infant–mother romance with the everyday: an early participation of reality in the otherwise narcissistic rapture of mutual love.

It is not only through the breast-feed that the mother conveys her erotism. She bathes the infant in seductive sonic imagery, ooing, cooing and aaahing, luring the infant's being from autistic enclave into desire for this voice. As the mother words her infant's gestures, with the onomatopoetics of 'ooing' and 'aaahing', she extends his or her body through this sonic imagery, which is maternal *parole*. If language is a third object derived from the patriarchal order (as John Muller eloquently argues,1996), one that divides selves from imaginary unity, maternal speech is acoustic signifier as body-ego action. Her speech attaches itself to the moving parts of the baby's body, driven by her affective sense of its requirements.

Maternal speech is more a thing presentation to the infant, composed of 'a complex of associations made up of the greatest variety of visual, acoustic, tactile, kinaesthetic and other presentations' (Freud 1915: 213). Only later will the meaning of 'these innumerable single impressions' (Freud 1917: 256) be linked to words, as they move from the deepest recesses of the unconscious into the preconscious and eventually into consciousness. (Indeed, it is not uncommon for adults who know the lyrics to a song to discover that they had never asked what the words mean, so taken were they by the sonic property of the words.) Maternal speech links language to desire long before words-in-themselves are used by the child to express desire. In 'voicing over' the infant's body, the mother touches her infant through acoustic fingers, precursive to all conversions from word to body, and likewise accomplishing its reversal, as the body is now put into words.

The cure of the hysteric depends on the patient 'getting his words in the 'right place': into sound, rather than allowing them to be caught up in his body', writes John Forrester (1990: 13), yet it is important to bear in mind that in the infant–mother relation sounds are caught up in the body. All hysterics are biased to keep the word in the body, as such conversions 'remember' a form of maternal erotism. As the mother's words, however, *substituted* for physical touch, the hysteric also seeks in the sonic imagery of the word the self's erotic body, so the transformational sequence of the cure must be from body to sound to signifier. The hysteric uses the word presentation as a thing presentation, transforming it into a direct impact of oneself upon the other's unconscious. The impish moves of the hysteric are meant to bring a smile to the other's face and an 'oooohhhh' or 'woooooowwww'. Vowel love opens the mouth wide and cracks up the face; it is preferable to consonants, which bear the knowledge of reality. The hysteric does not intend to take the word for what it means or conveys (in-itself), but for what it affects. It not only shows the body to the other, it is meant to enter the other's body as a shimmering palimpsest of excitation, engaging other thing presentations in the other's world, a kind of intercourse within the system unconscious.

Ironically, in a psychoanalysis, the very depth of such unconscious communication eventually dispossesses the hysteric of life inside the mother, as free associations produce a wealth of meanings which continually transfer the hysteric's imaginary into the symbolic, transferring life inside the maternal imaginary into a field of relations, intermediated by language. If language acquisition presents the self with the loss of maternal acoustic holding, then in the child who suffers the absence of maternal physical sanction of the self's embodied being, the loss is deeply painful, for in the thing-presentational effect of language is to be found maternal erotisation of the self's body.

As we shall discuss in a subsequent chapter, life in the maternal order – from a Freudian point of view – must be infant and mother affecting each other as impressions. Insofar as the infant is concerned, the unconscious will in the first place be composed of thing presentations, the traces of the self's experience of the mother. Indeed, in many respects, the relation between thing presentations – which constitute the primary repressed unconscious – *is* the psychical system between infant and mother. Thus not only is the unconscious formed out of the impact of the mother as thing, but the system unconscious sustains this mother within us for the remainder of our life. To understand the peculiar affliction and talent of hysterics, we must appreciate that they seek to live within a thing-presentational order, which in many respects constitutes their effort to usurp the symbolic order (itself linked to the father) with the power of the primary repressed system of unconscious communication. Very often this passion is the trace of maternal erotism.

The exception is the fate of the ascetic hysteric whose mother declines this erotisation and remains silent. If she nonetheless conveys her love of the infant as a being, but withholds celebration of the infant's sexuality, she passes on silence as the word. 'Shuuuuuusssssshhh. Mum's the word.' This silent mother is taken in as the self's silence, captured by the death drive.

The precocious hysteric is overworded by the mother, who, in reparative compensation, attaches her infant to the life instinct. Only later, when the hysteric is verbose, using words to theatric effect, does the hysteric sense the paradox of this loss: that in using words to evacuate his or her mental contents, the hysteric is emptied by his or her desire. Only in psychoanalysis is this loss remedied but at the cost of losing pure effect to uncertain meaning.

Let us return to maternal erotism.

A mother caresses her infant in countless ways. Whether she nibbles its ears, blows on its stomach, caresses its feet, or tousles its hair, she evokes the child's erotic capability. In the daily routine of nappy-changing and bathing she caresses the infant's genitals and anus, stimulating them through her own hands, accompanied by vocal, gestural and facial celebrations. Children return these festivities, squealing with delight, kicking their feet, or trying out the pleasures of speech.

Freud believed that the developing child must 'fuse' sexual and aggressive libido, a task which he saw as fundamentally intrapsychic. This task of bringing the two drives together is an ongoing intrapsychic function, but he omitted the mother's role in partnering sexuality and aggression, since through her enjoyment of the infant's sexuality and aggression she joins the instincts. The original fusion is through her hands. Lying on its back as the mother changes its nappy, the infant kicks her hand and squeals with delight. She returns the kick with her own aggression, shoving the foot back, perhaps saying 'Ah, so you want to make trouble for mama do you?', clearly celebrating the infant's aggressions. Every day, for years, she finds her child's sexual and aggressive bodily expressions delightful in countless ways, linking the drives and transferring the very body she has aroused into language.

When we imagine the mother of the hysteric, however, we come across a somewhat different figure. My speculation will oversimplify her further, as the scene to be described need not be behaviourally dramatic, but could be very subtle indeed. Further, a good-enough mother, capable of the celebrations described above, may be temporarily disabled, or the child, armed against embodied being, may refuse maternal desire.

One mother, for example, recalled how the death of her own mother coincided with the birth of her second child. So grief-stricken that she could not celebrate his birth, he was to suffer as a result, unlike her other children, whom she enjoyed. Another mother could never understand why she disliked her third child's body, so unlike that of her other three children: 'I just took one look at it after its birth and there was something about it which was repelling. I thought to myself that it was a mistake and that this was not my child.' For years she was aware that she could not enjoy this child's bodily being, although her remove was very subtle, not dramatic, and she struggled with her ambivalence in private and in psychoanalysis. Another mother had her first child of several just as she discovered that her husband was having an affair. Her child was a boy. She could not look at his body, especially the penis, without feeling enraged with men for letting their pricks guide their destiny. She said once: 'I held his body with rage in my hands.' Another mother felt that no matter how she cuddled and stroked her infant there was always some strange detachment in the baby, leaving her feeling that her desire was unrequited.

There are countless reasons, then, why certain women under certain circumstances simply cannot celebrate their infants' bodies. Along with these, there is another mother who communicates much the same dilemma, and, not surprisingly, she is hysteric. I can think of no better way to introduce this type of mother than to provide an account from one of my patients.

> I had for years thought that I would have a child, because for me it was a natural act of fulfilment. I enjoyed my younger brothers and sisters and as I am a bit of a child myself, I longed for the time when I could just hang out in the home with them. I love the word 'mum' and I wanted to hear myself addressed in this way. Although I did worry about how I would have the time for this, given my work, I reckoned that with proper organisation and child care it would work out. I imagined weekends with the kids. As time passed and I got married it became more pressing, not only because I was now in my mid-thirties, but also because something physically near by was missing in my relation to my husband. We had never been sexually close, although we were companionable, and I wanted warm cuddly bodies to look after and snuggle up with.
>
> When I became pregnant I read all the books on childbirth and thought I would be ready for it all, and in some ways I was. I did not reckon on quite how long and hard the labour would be – it was fifteen hours – and I suppose

like a lot of women it was something of a shock. There is a difference between the literary experience and the actual experience! Anyway, that was not to be the problem. What happened next was just very surprising, to some extent embarrassing, but mostly heartbreaking. That is, looking back on it. At the time I think I denied the problem. Which was, that although I was enormously pleased to have given birth to a little girl, and although I was absolutely thrilled with the way she looked, and her simple little gestures, and wonderful particularities, I was totally shocked to see her vagina looking as it did. I should have known it would look as it did; in fact, I'm sure I knew. I am sure I had seen other infant girls. What I saw looked like an enormous open wound, a huge gash, and it was the size of it – in comparison to the rest of the body – which also seemed to me to be what was so horrible about it.

Anyway, whenever bathing her in the months to come, I had to avert my gaze rather than touch it. I remember trying all sorts of wiping techniques to go over it without sensing it, so to speak. So sometimes I would wipe her up from the anus in one fell swoop, moving up to the navel. But of course that was unhygienic. Then I found rather large fluffy cloths made in China which I used to cover most of that part of the body. And although I loved touching her hands or her feet, loved looking at her face, and kissing her cheeks, whenever I had to touch her genitals, my hands changed. I was either stiff, or too quick, or too officious. This is in looking back. At the time, I think I just denied it, although I gradually knew that I did not know what to do with her vagina.

Time passed and I thought it had to do with her being a girl. But then I had a son and much the same problem arose again. I did not know how to touch his penis and did so stiffly or unlovingly, and there were times when I just dreaded the entire enterprise. The strange thing is that I don't think I even knew what the problem was. Or that there was any problem. I think I originally thought of the situation in terms of my just being too harassed with duties and this was one more duty I had to perform. So I think I just put it down to being overworked.

What this woman describes seems to me a clear statement of the problem a mother can have with her baby's body, one that will be communicated to the infant, and which would constitute a predisposition to hysteria. Later she elaborated her perceptions, recalling that her daughter's vagina seemed huge and swollen and that she experienced her son's penis as 'having a life of its own'. When it became erect, she said, she thought that it might detach itself from his body; she corrected this to say; 'once I wished it would just "go away", jump off and leave. Then I imagined that like a mouse it might be in hiding and I accepted it was better that it remain attached to his body. These were sort of "crazy ideas" which were curiously pleasing.'

Specifically, the mother experiences intense ambivalence towards the infant as a sexual being, especially towards the genitalia, which cannot be sensorially celebrated. Maternal care is in this respect a 'laying on of hands' and the mother in this case cannot eroticise her infant's body through her own hands. From this perspective we would have to conclude that the original paralysis that enervates the hysteric comes through an enervation of maternal touch. We may speculate that the mother communicates this ambivalence towards the infant who will, however, know of this message only through a correspondent enervation of the genitalia as love objects, although these mothers may try to make it up by celebrating other parts of the infant's body – such as the face, the feet, the shoulders, the stomach, the back – which become alternative erotic zones: displacements – enacted now by the mother – that may serve as subsequent conduits of excitation.

It is important to note that, in theory, we now have an interlinking network of several of the key constituents known to feature in the formation of hysteria:

1   *repression* (of maternal excitation);
2   its *transmission* to the infant;
3   by way of *conversion* to the infant's body;
4   through an *enervation* of the mother's touch;
5   mitigated by *displacement* of the genital–sexual to the non-genital erotic zones of the body, lighting it up like a Christmas tree with flashing desire;
6   further compensated by *passing the word* into the body, where it is meant to retain its status as a thing presentation;
7   leading the infant to *identify* with an other who finds the sexual self unacceptable.

The mother described on pp. 45–47 found her infant's genitals sexually repelling, but she did attempt breast-feeding, finding it acceptable up to a point, before she retreated from erotic reverie. The degree of maternal ambivalence is an important factor in the predisposition of the infant. If the mother finds breast-feeding unacceptably sexual and withdraws her cathexis of the infant's desire, then she will convey this to the baby. She may elect to avoid breast-feeding altogether.

The breast is the erotic epicentre of the self's relation to the other, and certainly the precursor of the genital, which will follow it many years later as the axis of desire between self and other. It is from the breast that excitation radiates through the body as deep being, from mouth into body and through its total being.

If the mother then refuses the infant's genital sexuality – not sonically celebrating it, averting her gaze, stiffening her touch – thereby displacing it to the other parts of the body – now serving as microepicentres of a decentred sexuality – she has removed the core of erotic life and sought surface sexuality as a defence against deep sexuality. Her wording joins this decentred sexuality as her vocal celebrations of the non-genital parts are captured by the erotogenic area which the word signifies: 'Oh! . . . what . . . big feet!', if serving as displaced representatives of the uncelebrated genital, link word to body and bury both in a shallow grave, skin deep.

This exchange (genitals for the remaining parts of the body) predisposes the child to an hysteric's management of sexual excitation, as the body becomes unusually charged with displaced libido.[1] In foreplay, therefore, hysterics often find the arousal of the non-genital erotogenic zones exquisitely compelling, yet this bliss is at the same time the source of a depressive rage, as the genital self[2] is to be refused. The self will be in early mourning, as hysteric-style erotism avoids core ecstasy, and genital aversion unconsciously recalls the refusals of the breast. The child feeds on tertiary excitations aimed to distract it from core erotism, a displacement that saturates the child's desire with unconscious grief.

Many people can recall the mother's erotic link to a displaced part of the body. A patient recollects his mother's back rubs as sensual if unusual.

> My mother was a wonderful and vivid person but ordinarily she would not touch me. By that I mean that she would never hug me – even if we hadn't seen each other for a long time. She would convey delight by giggling and immediately talking about what she had just then been doing, such as gardening, but she would not engage in physical contact. Only when she was quite elderly would she let me kiss her on the cheek, which I think she was surprised to discover as more pleasant than she knew. But there was one amazing exception. When I was a boy and even up to early adolescence, she would rub my back. When I was very young she would do it at bedtime when she would say 'turn over, I will rub your back' – and she would give me long rubs that would put me off to sleep. It wasn't until I was an adult that I realised that when I visited grandmother she would do the very same thing, and so I assume that this is where my mother got it. It was the only permitted form of sensual pleasure between my mother and myself.

This may be simply another variety of the body as signifier, something so crucial to Freud's study of the hysteric and to the classical theory of conversion. If so, the body is already undergoing conversion experiences in this first relation, as the mother represses her relation to the genital and finds another part of the body to function in its place.

As maternal love is the first field of sexual foreplay, the hysterical mother conveys to her infant's body an anguished desire, as her energetic touches bear the trace of disgust and frustration, carrying to the infant's body communications about sexual ambivalence, 'rolfed', as it were, into the infant's body knowledge, part of the self's unthought known.[3]

In 'On narcissism: an introduction' (1914) Freud writes that an organ's 'erotogenicity' is an 'activity of sending sexually exciting stimuli to the mind' and that certain 'erotogenic zones . . . may act as substitutes for the genitals and behave analogously to them'. But a characteristic of the genital is that 'it becomes congested with blood, swollen and humected, and is the seat of a multiplicity of sensations' (p. 84); so for other organs to be 'analogous' to the genital they must either become congested with excitation in this manner, or behave as if they were. It is in stimulating the infant's mouth, eyes, ears, feet, stomach, etc. to the point of swelling with excitement that the mother displaces her genital interests into non-genital excitational equivalents. This is perhaps the moment to point out that so-called eating disorders involve a swelling and emptying of the body (the anorectic believes the body is swollen with too much fat), ideas which are partly generated by the dread of the body's sexuality, which is sexualised as an illness of swelling up and slimming down.

As the mother hypercathects the non-gential erotogenic zones, she unconsciously distributes the child's erotism over the surface of the body, radiating in intensity away from the genital. If genital erotism (and eventually genital intercourse) involves sexual depth – literally, in penetrating into the other or in being penetrated – hysterical erotism sexualises the surface in order to avoid sexual depth.

It is of interest that many so-called body therapies involve a laying-on of hands, and we may wonder whether some of the intense popularity of these treatments is partly due to the self's finding a form of body confirmation. Being touched by the other – in differing forms of massage or body therapies – may well be a paradigmatic cure by the hands of the other. Ironically, however, such treatments sometimes stimulate a craving that cannot (ordinarily) be supplied, as this laying-on of hands is not meant to be erotic, leaving the client in a type of ongoing dependence upon repeated treatments. If the individual is hysteric then body therapy joins the primary object in declining the erotic needs of the self, especially as this therapy caresses only the surface of the body and does not ordinarily become intercourse.

There is, as one can imagine, an extraordinarily wide spectrum of maternal responses to an infant's body. The more ordinary ambivalent states resemble those described in the above account of a mother's failure to enjoy her infant's genitals (pp. 45–47); we may assume that her attitude toward the child's sexual body is very subtly one of declining an invitation of sorts. Some mothers, on the other hand, are openly disapproving of their infant's genitalia and regard cleaning the genitals as 'dirty work', which must nevertheless be carried out. Others regard the child's masturbatory genital offerings as 'nasty' and tell the girl not to spread her legs and show the vagina, or the boy not to show his penis.

Maternal ambivalence toward the infant's sexuality takes the form of a negative hallucination, rimming the genitals with maternal blindness. A patient explains this best.

> I am having a hard time these days, there are things which I should tell you but which are not so easy. I find myself just staring at [my infant boy] or glaring . . . or, well, I find that I look at his penis. It is an odd object, by all accounts. I absolutely do not know what I think about it. It is strange that it, or rather that he, came out of my body. It doesn't have anything to do with me, I think, and yet it does. But I am being too . . . a bit aside from the point . . . I think that my mood changes in relation to it, or rather, that I have different feelings about it, wildly different feelings. There are days, or rather, moments when I think it is great, it's an amazing sight, and I am pleased to see it; then in a few seconds

> I can feel that it is ugly, disgraceful, and completely 'unnecessary': that's the word that crosses my mind. I know I convey something of this to [the boy] because when I bath him, sometimes I talk to him about his penis in a good way – you know – saying things like 'what a strong boy', or 'what a nice penis'; but then, there are times when I feel that he is showing it off to me and I feel like cutting it off, I just feel cold, and indifferent. Well . . . not indifferent. I actually feel like I hate it. But it stirs up the most intense feelings at the time. I've no idea what he is making of this.

Nor do we. But this patient illuminates in consciousness what resides in differing intensities in the unconscious of all mothers, notably, that ambivalence which all of us possess in relation to the genital. Unlike the mother who could not look at her infant's genitals, this mother is absorbed in them. She later described a wide range of expressed affects in relation to her son's penis. She would chortle, or laugh, or reproach him, or feel depressed and convey it. We could say that she would blow hot and cold, feeling passionate love and equally passionate repulsion.

When Freud treated Frau Cacile M he noted her unusually developed 'sense of form' (Breuer and Freud 1893: 180) revealed in her poetry. This leads him to discuss hysterical symptomatology, when the hysteric 'creates a somatic expression for an emotionally-coloured idea by symbolisation' (p. 180), which, he concludes, has less to do with 'personal' or 'voluntary factors' than it does with the fundamental link between a word and the body. When the hysteric expresses a verbal expression 'literally', such as feeling 'a stab in the heart' or 'a slap in the face' after a slight, the hysteric is 'not taking liberties with words, but is simply revealing once more the sensations to which the verbal expression owes its justification' (p. 181). Freud concludes that the phrase 'stabbed in the heart' must owe itself to a moment when the person feels 'a precordial sensation which could suitably be described' by this term. Equally, finding something 'hard to swallow' betrays the link between word and body, because such an expression would originate, he believes, from 'innervatory sensations which arise in the pharynx when we refrain from speaking and prevent ourselves from reacting to an insult' (p. 181).

As the mother voices over her infant's body she forges links between word and body. We see this effect in films of depressed mothers with their infants, as the mother – trying to be of some assistance to her infant – cannot help but word the child as an extension of her depression: Lynn Murray's films, for example, often show a mother handing an object to the infant with the words 'poor love' or 'poor baby' passed to the infant's psyche-soma.

Among the variations in hysterical mothering, then, is the mother who charges her words with erotic anxiety or erotic ambivalence, conveyed to her infant as she voices over his or her existence. As we will discuss in the next chapter, she may bias her child toward precocious identifications, with the language of sexuality as a form of manic transcendence over engaged sexuality; whilst the mother who employs a negative hallucination may bias her child toward the psychology of transcendence through abstinence. These categories are not, however, as distinct or irrevocable as one might think, since both positions nonetheless bear signs of maternal anguish over the child's reproductive fate. In addition, the child who sets against his or her maturational process an expression of the death instinct, may decline erotic reciprocity with the mother, choosing schizoid erotism: the cathexis of voice or vision as removed alternative to engaged sensuality.

It is important to bear in mind, however, that for the most part the sort of maternal processes described above are not equivalent to maternal hate of the child's very being. These mothers are women who decline to celebrate their children's sexuality. At this stage in our considerations we shall be discussing a mother who loves her infant and who, to differing degrees, is disturbed by her difficulty with the infant's genitals and sexual gestures. If she is herself an hysteric, then she will take evasive action through an alternative form of loving. In talking and showing, or in narrative and performance, she will find a setting in which she can love her son or her daughter. To some extent, telling and showing the infant one's love of them is an ordinary part of any mother's mothering, but with the woman who finds her infant's sexuality repelling, her guilt and her need to make reparation intensify the significance of narrating and performing this love.

Furthermore, the infant she celebrates in the erotics of voice, or caresses in the sexuality of gaze or in the dramatic performance of her body's delight over the infant's body, is one step removed from the infant. Thus she does not engage the actual body but sets about vigorously cathecting its imaginary twin. Like it or not, the infants of hysterical mothers share her with an imaginary companion, perhaps first offered by the mother as her love object.

As we shall discuss in Chapter 9, the hysteric shows off the self, transforming it into an event ready for inspection by the other. This stance expresses the self's arrest, or fixation, at the point when mother's language and child's sexuality are meant to fuse, in the acquisition of words that one can live with and which are psychically transformative. The hysteric shows us that he or she cannot accept the link between the body's expressed sexuality and the other's worded desire of it. It must be shown again and again. We see this simple fact in the young boy or girl taking a bath, spreading the legs to display the penis or the vagina to the mother, with what seems like a curiously knowing look in their smiling face. What does the mother say to this? How does this showing off move into language?

As long as the hysteric presents the body as a non-genital sexualised delight, he or she can link his or her bodily being with maternal desire. But the genital pulsion evokes unconscious memories of maternal repulsion and will remain fundamentally unprocessed. As the mother relates to the infant's genital with a dead hand, she declines both to celebrate it and to word it, thus leaving genital excitation untransformed. It is of interest that the hysteric suffers an excess of non-genital erotic transformations, often verging on a kind of exhibitionist theatre, but when it comes to the genital moment the self is suddenly and dramatically an infantile creature with no sense of erotic destiny. Indeed, whilst the erogenous zones that do allow for the hysteric's erotism are occasions for display and receptive transmission, such contact points also double as zones of eventual sorrow.

We will return to this topic later. For now, we are left to contemplate the functions of maternal narrative, which are unusually overdetermined in the case of the hysteric. In a certain respect, narrative takes the place of hands-on mothering. In the course of the child's development he or she will be a lively figure inside maternal narrative as she talks to the child about all the facets of life, including their relation, a telling which is libidinalised through an exchange of desire from the actual to the narrative, or from the real to the imaginary. Often enough, especially in good pairings of mother and child, the child will become a storyteller, enjoying narrative as a kind of collaborative alternative to possible actual experiences, especially those involving certain sexual engagements.

From this ordinary aspect of maternal care, and the evolution of the self's internal world, the child constructs the theory that he or she is also alive in the silent chambers of the mother's internal world: especially in her reveries. For it will also be in one's own reveries that the self communes with actual others as internal object.

Ordinary reveries of this sort may, however, have to substitute for the relative absence of the sensorial and erotic being of the other; ironically, this too is projected into the primary object, similarly engaged with internal erotic objects at the comparative expense of the actual others who are ready at hand.

An example from adult life may help. A young woman sought psychotherapy after the failure of her third love relation. It became clear that when she and a lover were in bed she wanted him just to talk about life and their relation before 'doing anything'. She needed something like an hour or more, during which she felt that through exchanging stories of their lives and of the events of the day, she could then make love. No sooner had this taken place than she wanted to talk to her lover about what it had been like for him and to talk and talk about other matters that came to mind. I gathered from her descriptions that if love-making took about three hours, the actual time spent in foreplay and intercourse was about ten minutes, with the remaining hours spent talking. All her lovers had expressed frustration with her demand to talk. She in turn felt that they were insensitive and too brutally insistent upon having their own way. It was quite some time before she understood that for her, talking and narrating was the livelier place of sexual life than the act of love-making itself. Fortunately, she was not in deep hostility to her sexuality and could discover, over time, that she and her lovers could talk to their hearts' content in the proper contexts and not as unconscious evasions of realised desire.

She was unaware of the fact that she needed to convert actual others into internal objects, and that her sharing of lengthy narrative with her lovers was a way of turning them first into narrative objects – and hearing where the self resided in the lover's narrative world – and then into erotically residing internal objects, so that in the brief flash of love-making, the evoked internal object and the actual other momentarily fused. One of her lovers commented on the oddity of this moment, when he said that although she seemed unusually reticent to make love and seemed uncomfortable with being touched – uncertain, sort of jumpy and jerky – in the moment of orgasm she had a possessed look on her face, as if she had found a place she had been seeking for a long time. This differs from the loss of consciousness of normal orgasm in that normal orgasm is a dispossession of the fantastic by the emergent power of the engagements of erotic knowledge, as we will discuss in a later chapter. The hysteric, by contrast, disappears into the auto-erotic object at the moment it touches the real, as when the above patient accepted her lover's body and sexuality just as it finally converged with the imaginary object of desire.

Living inside the other's narrative.

One of Freud's first reported hysterics (1895), Frau Emmy von N, lived inside stories that she then narrated and/or performed for Freud. On 1 May 1889 – the day he first meets her – he finds her 'lying on a sofa with her head resting on a leather cushion' (p. 48): inventing the analytical position before it has become standard posture. On the second day Freud speculates that 'it is safe to suppose that she has read about hypnotism' (p. 51) as she takes to it so readily, and on 8 May she 'entertained' him with 'gruesome stories about animals' that 'she had read in the *Frankfurter Zeitung*' (p. 51). A boy had died of fright when an apprentice put a white mouse to his mouth. Emmy narrates this, but in a moment she performs it for Freud: 'She clenched and unclenched her hand several times. "Keep still! – Don't say anything! – Don't touch me! – Supposing a creature like that was in the bed!" (She shuddered)' (p. 51). (Interestingly, Freud misses this transference reference, as at other moments he had been massaging Emmy and giving her baths. But true to his developing comprehension of the hysteric, it is of interest that both should miss the significance of his touch – at least so far as we know, since *it* goes unnarrated – whilst self and other find stories to get inside. Thus both move *from* body to narrative. Also, 'ruhe!' means not only 'no excitement' but also 'Don't say anything', referring this couple to the supposed refuge of maternal silence.)

Freud wipes away her memories during hypnosis, a common process of abreactive technique, but 'whilst she was asleep I picked up the *Frankfurter Zeitung*' (p. 51) to discover that the story did not contain references to mice or rats: these Emmy had supplied herself. Patient and analyst have entered the narrative of the other, there to find some truth that generates identifications.

That evening Freud returns and Emmy narrates memories from her childhood; Freud writes that 'at the end of each separate story she twitched all over and took on a look of fear and horror' (p. 53) The next morning, 9 May, she recalls that her governess had 'brought her an ethnological atlas and that some pictures in it of American Indians dressed up as animals had given her a great shock' (p. 53). As she thinks about it, she is frightened by the pictures and Freud tries to calm her. That evening she recalls that a maidservant who had once worked for a mistress who had been in an asylum 'used to tell her horrifying stories' (p. 55), which Emmy proceeds to show and tell.

As Emmy continues to tell stories about memories and stories told by others, Freud aims to remove such scenes from her mind – perhaps unconsciously trying to restore to the hysteric a type of benign blank screen that will allow thought to proceed from within the self, rather than leave the self besieged by what it hears or sees – but he does not fathom the structure of the hysteric's transmission: that of a self caught up in the stories of the other, bound to identify with them, and then to narrate and perform them. All along, as we are to discover, Emmy's grimaces and distorted facial representations bear her identification with her mother's death mask (at 19 Emmy came home one day and found her mother dead, with a distorted face) – a mother who had also apparently been in an asylum, and who, I imagine, very probably cathected the child as a narrative and performative object.

Freud takes part in reading the self's place inside the other. 'I gradually came to be able to read from patients' faces', he writes, 'whether they might not be concealing an essential part of their confessions' (1895d: 79) This reflection is an expression of what much later would be termed the countertransference, as the patient situates the analyst in a direct unconscious relation to the patient's predicament. Freud, like the hysteric, develops an unconscious expertise in detecting a story by reading the face of the other. Yet unlike Emmy, who will then identify with the contents of the story and either narrate or perform it before the other, Freud chooses to write up what he sees and to pass it on as literature. Still, such transmission as a form of hysteria cannot pass without comment, and Freud's final footnote to this case – written in 1924 – is telling: 'I am aware that no analyst can read this case history today without a smile of pity' (p. 105). How ironic, however, that he does not note how close he comes in such a moment to his own position when listening to the pathos narrated by Emmy. What will be made, he wonders, by the listening (or reading) other who hears a subject's account of being captivated by a compelling other? And how interesting it is that Freud's imagined reader combines the narrative and the performative moment, or the verbal and the visual: for this reader shows a smile upon the face.

As they discover that important libidinal relations which could have been expressed more openly in the actual relations to the self are now sustained within the maternal internal world – expressed now and then in her narratives and in her live action performances – hysterics become anxious to know who they are to the other. In all subsequent relations, they have the knack of invading the other to find out who they are to that other, and this has often led the hysteric to be mis-diagnosed as a borderline personality, because there is a certain type of boundary violation. Such break-ins aim to discover the self's status as the other's secret object of desire, whereas the borderline invasion creates in mutual distress a shared object, bonding both people in a borderline frame of mind.

The hysteric's solution to the question 'what has happened to my sexuality?' results in the development of two inseparable skills. As the answer to this question resides in the other's internal world, the hysteric seeks to enter that world to find the particular objects of maternal desire. Once that object is constructed, the hysteric then tries to identify with it and then to represent it to the mother. These skills – identification and representation – can be developed to a remarkable degree by hysterics, who show uncanny abilities to gain access to the other's desire and then to represent it. Whether one chooses to say, therefore, that the hysteric is always the maternal phallus – and thus acting out the phallus from the maternal imaginary – or that the hysteric is the maternal self object – or any other object of maternal desire – these acts are always self-sacrificial. The hysteric abandons his or her true self in order to substitute it with the supposed object of maternal desire. In place of the self's presentation of its idiom, carried forth in the countless ordinary acts of everyday life without much thought, is the self's presentation of the other's object of desire, a highly mediated form of re-presentation, bearing with it anxiety over the delivery and mourning over the cost.

Hysterics demonstrate what we might think of as the moment of self disruption, when the true self is abandoned for a type of false orientation to the object world. Psychoanalysts working with hysterics note how these patients may suddenly say out of the blue, 'So what do you think?' or 'You said that I was competitive, so does that mean you see me as some kind of dragoness?' They momentarily dissociate themselves from the previously associative collaborations with the analyst. In stepping back, they invite the analyst into his or her assumed maternal hysteria, to expose the analyst's concept of the patient. This internal object would then become the passionate object of desire, shared between the two participants. The borderline seeks to elicit the analyst's anguish, joining both in mutual rage and in dismay. The hysteric seeks a dissociative space into which is inserted an imaginary figure of desire, which can serve as play object for both.

Hysterics may seek out details about the analyst's private life in order to infer who they are to the analyst. The borderline analysand, however, will be invasive and persecuting, because in creating distress within the analyst, the patient and the analyst share the primary object together. The hysteric is charming and beguiling – and the analyst is very often mentally inclined to disclose private thoughts of an affectionate type – whereas the borderline is persecuting and infuriating – the analyst is in a defensive frame of mind.

Still, as the hysteric does not know from maternal touch what the other desires, there is an anxious need to have evidence of one's erotic appeal. This may lead the hysteric to over-intense, somewhat invasive, forays into the analyst's inner life (or private life) in the effort to extract evidence of the analyst's desire.

The hysteric has also been the object of a certain type of maternal cancellation of the self's desire, and this erasure lives on as a type of blankness or absence that bears the trace of its originating aggression: where 'it' once was, there shall cancellation be. Oftentimes the hysteric will bring the clinician up short by curtly saying 'I have no idea', or 'Not a clue' to a question about what is on his or her mind. These sudden erasures are all the more telling if the two people have been enjoying a certain type of rapport. For example, one analysand would typically put a damper on our work, when about mid-way through an hour she would say 'What do you mean?' or 'Could you go over that again?' These would almost always be rather stunning occasions, all the more puzzling as the manifest content was clear and not confusing. She invited me to move from psychic collaboration to cognition proper, from more unconscious forms of work to hyper-extended forms of consciousness. She would go back over the contents of the session and tell me what it had been like for her to have experienced the hour. Often she would stitch together parts of the session and previous sessions into a tapestry that seemed almost wilfully persecutory. By so distorting our understandings of one another, she tried to goad me into joining her in telling her my 'version' of what we had been talking about in the hour, or in previous sessions. I said she seemed to invite the two of us into becoming storytellers, with her telling me a tale about the two of us, inviting me to do the same. As we had long since already discussed how important it was for her to narrate her life to people – in that everyone who meant anything to her had to listen to endlessly repeated stories of her distant and recent past – it was now possible to show her how she was inviting the two of us to live separate lives, out of touch with each other, just swapping stories of the other's changing status within, as an internal object of the self's wayward thoughts.

Are there differences in the boy's and the girl's sexual resolutions of maternal rejection of the self's sexuality? In a certain limited sense, yes. The boy can take refuge in the self's sexual difference to sustain an unconscious notion that his difference automatically makes for a different route to sexual destiny. The girl would be more likely to suffer the unconscious fate of assuming that, as she and the mother share the same gender, the maternal interpretation of the girl's sexuality would automatically be definitive. Sameness of gender would suggest sameness of sexual life, sameness of psychic life. But as we know, girls and women struggle throughout a lifetime against these communications and the fantasies to which they give rise, so much so, that we may observe an irony in this journey: that the woman may actually have achieved greater differentiation from the mother's unconscious than the man, whose assumptions of difference lessen his struggle to define himself, and lull him into a less clear sense of himself.

The problem with gender-categorical thinking, however, is the problem of the individual case. One simply finds too many exceptions to these grand schemes of things and, as discussed in Chapter 2, an individual's sexuality is not equivalent to his or her gender. A man could develop a negative Oedipus complex, making love in the unconscious to his father, yet he could be a manifest heterosexual with wife and children. He could live out his sexuality by taking pleasure in buying tickets for male companions to football games, or he could be a camp counsellor, hiring famous athletes to come and teach the children. If we wished to make this more complex, and thus do a better job of indicating how overdetermined human sexuality is, we could add that his negative Oedipus complex is in fact an identification with his father's negative complex – i.e. his father's love of his father – with which our subject is identified. Let's make it more complex still. Let's imagine that our subject's supposed unconscious homosexuality – a passionate disposition to service other men – which puts him in the female position, is his grandfather's solution to the death of his mother. Thus the patient's father has handed down to him his own father's grief over loss of the mother, so that homosexuality here is intended to make up for the disappearance of the mother. And it gets much more complex than this. At the end, when we seek to schematise human sexuality under the banner of gender, we subject any self to an over-simplification that does not stand the test of psychoanalytical investigation.

Returning to the hysteric, then, we cannot assume an automatic psychic disposition in the girl. She might or she might not find sexual sameness a determining issue in her life. Her brother might find himself in intense identification with his mother's body, so much more than herself, that he has a harder time in life sorting out his own self from the mother's self. Indeed, the core issue of hysteria is both genders' sense that the mother has withdrawn her love of the self's genitalia. Although, ostensibly, this would seem to be – so far as the child is concerned – withdrawal of her validation of the child's gender, inseparable from the genital, in fact, the mother conveys her disgust with all genitals: male or female. The mother is sexually democratic, treating the girl and the boy with equal disgust, just as she finds in her own vagina and in her husband's penis equal zones of repulsion.

It is best to limit the prescriptive theatre of psychoanalytic role creation as much as possible. But I have imagined a mother, I have given her a mythic place, and I have assigned her a particular role in relation to her infant. I walk a thin line between referring to the prescription imposed by character restriction – that is, the self-defining limits of the hysteric character – and imposing a role upon this actual person. We must keep this in mind as we turn now to another story, the tale of the hysteric's father. I believe this story to be true, but I also know it is constructed out of my own and other psychoanalysts' imaginations as we create theory in order to think about our patients.

I am of course aware of the irony of this moment: in discussing how the hysteric seeks to exist inside the other's story I am creating one of my own, which could become an open house for any travelling hysteric. It could not be otherwise.

The solution to this paradox is for the psychoanalyst to make his or her theory of hysteria lucidly clear to the patient in sessions. All patients will comprehend this as the analyst's perspective and its strengths, such as they are, will reveal themselves in the hysteric's gradual integration of his or her genital sexuality and the correspondent pleasure in rejoining the maturational process. How do we know this is not an act of compliance? How do we know that the hysteric has not read our desire – in this case the theory of hysteria – and is now determined to supply it? The answer is that the hysteric will always do this, under all circumstances. In one respect, however, the hysteric's fulfilment of the analyst's desire is the fulfilment of the desire that the patient return to being his or her own true self. How?

The analyst seeks to place the patient before what we might call the open object, functioning as a medium for the self's articulation of its unconscious life. The hysteric who simply fulfils the copy of the analyst's desire will not achieve unconscious freedom in the analytical hour. Only through free association will the analysand reveal the extent of liberation from the analyst's desire, accomplished in his or her thick movement in the symbolic order, to which even the analysand is not in the know. In unconscious freedom the self is disseminated through the free play of affects, images, words and relational positions, whilst in states of compliance the analysand seeks to mirror the analyst's interpretations or indirectly so, by proposing a reliable opposition to them which accomplishes compliance through predictable counter-dependent action.

Even as the hysteric resists the analyst's storytelling, hearing who one is to the analyst is pleasurable. For some time, it shall be to the pleasure of patient and analyst to tell this story. Eventually, however, the sets of interpretations will become tedious. The analyst will be disinclined to make them. Both will turn to other matters and this is how it must be. If this book is about the right length, then the reader will be tiring of it as he or she approaches the last pages, and want to get on with other readings by other writers. One hopes, then, for the natural decathexis of this story – for patient and for reader – after it has served its purpose.

The analyst must analyse the paradox of his place: that as an interpretive authority of sorts, the analyst infantilises the patient and thereby fulfils the hysteric's desire. The patient must eventually *take over* the interpretive process, which must be assimilated by the clinician's continued analysis of hysterical compliance. By the end of this person's analysis the hysteric structure recedes enough for the patient to enjoy the diversity of conflicted states of mind – psychotic, neurotic, normal – and the merciful pleasures of psychic sleeping: the ever-recurring intermissions of mental quiet.

It is in psychic sleeping that a self hatches, sponsors and cultivates unconscious creativity, such as preparing the night's dream, or working on an essay before a topic is known, or . . .

To return to where we left off, the story-in-itself will always function as the body of the mother, a constant lure for any hysteric. If, as discussed in Chapter 2 when quoting Sir Thomas Wyatt, hysterical passion is a conversion of carnal excitement into the ecstasy of self sacrifice – where the self shall now be a soul seeking its soul mate, but from a distance – the story-in-itself becomes an erotic place where this self can exist. Discussing Sidney's *Arcadia*, C.S. Lewis relates a story from Lucy Hutchinson's memoir of her husband: that is, a story told to her husband, which she passed on and which influenced Sidney!

> He told him of a gentleman who not long before found all the people bewailing the death of a gentlewoman that had lived there, and grew so in love with the description that he grew desperately melancholy and would goe to a mount where the print of her foote was cutt and lie there pining and kissing of it all the day long, till at length death concluded his languishment.
>
> (1944: 331)

Lewis wonders if 'many readers may ask whether the reality is not as foolish and tasteless as the fiction' (p. 331), contrasting this event with many fictional alternatives. But the erotism of the hysteric is in fact to move actual life into the realms of the story; so when the above gentleman heard the story of a gentlewoman's death, he was not simply captivated by the story, he turned his life into a figure who would inevitably attenuate and indeed enter the story. He entered her, as it were, through the ear of those hearing the tale, and now through the reader's eye; and he knew it. As we shall discuss in the final chapter, hysterics enter the other's story, there to dedicate, if not sacrifice, their life; and no literature is of more interest to them than stories written by psychoanalysts. They have been satisfying psychoanalysts' desire before analysts knew for whom they were looking and in what form. That irony must never elude the psychoanalyst who presumes to write about the hysteric.

We cannot conclude this chapter, however, without discussing the hysteric's presentation of the self to hospitals. The photographs and drawings of the hysteric collapsing in Charcot's arms seem to form an indelible image of the hysteric's suffering. It is as if the couch was invented to catch the hysteric's falling body. To this day, hysterics continue to present themselves to doctors and hospitals, under the pretext of a bodily ailment, at best to serve up a new-found illness, or at worst to have a part of their body removed unnecessarily. If we understand this presentation, however, as partly a transferential expression of the self's wish to have the body-as-ailment presented to the loving other (the doctor now being a figure who tends to bodies out of love), then we may comprehend the hysteric's constant visits to hospital as a continual call to the mother to take the self back into care, and to rediscover the infant's body as something now desirable.

We may see, then, that the hysteric's demi-erotic transference to the doctor, which may worry the hospital staff for its seeming impropriety, is indeed the reason for the visits and the search for a cure. Of course, the doctor cannot provide what the hysteric seeks, but disparagement of the hysteric for wasting valuable medical or hospital time is misguided: the patient's presentation of a false body ailment in order to use the body as the occasion for love is an astonishingly accurate use of the hospital by this person. All along the body suffered no intrinsic illness; it was purely a matter of the mother's rejection of the self's sexuality. When he or she is pleased to have an ailment confirmed as real, possibly even to have some small surgery, the hysteric feels that he or she will be the recipient of the doctor's intelligent love. Casting aside the paradox of a love that would remove a part of the body – in the unconscious always the genital – the hysteric finds in the surgeon's attentions a hand that seems so much more alive to the body's needs than that of the mother.

Anyway, the hysteric will turn to hospital as the place for the repeated presentation of the body. In so doing, he or she unconsciously seeks to undo the course of hysteria, even if, ironically enough, the surgeon's knife seems to inherit the maternal repression. In arriving for psychoanalysis, to drape the self on the couch, the hysteric re-presents the body that needs to be seen and interpreted again. Although the patient will resist references to this body, the fact is that psycho-analysis, in part, would appear to be the place for the privileging of the body in abject state. Will the psychoanalyst revive the Sleeping Beauty latent to this body so draped? Even as the analytical cure is by talking, the reality of hysteria is that the patient knows of psychoanalysis as a scene, as a picture of a self's embodied affliction presented to the eyes of the other. The analyst's wordings will be taken as forms of touching, caresses of the hysteric's other body, the body disincarnated into soul. Through the analyst's wordings of the patient's repressed desires, not only is the content of the hysteric's repressed returned to consciousness, but the underlying form of the repression – maternal refusal of the self's sexuality – is transformed by the analyst, who seeks to name and identify the self's sexuality. The hysteric's resistance to this process will always be two-fold. It will express the patient's alarm that the analyst is removing the patient from his or her Madonna–mamma, but discovery of the pleasure in wording sexuality returns the hysteric to forms of embodiment not previously experienced, and this fulfilment in the transference creates an unconscious vision of a new maternity and its new-born.

The hysteric's new birth takes place through the symbolic order, as it will be through talking that a new mother is implicitly arranged. Intriguingly, however, the symbolic order accomplishes a *Nachträglichkeit* upon the imaginary and the real; the after-effect of wording the hysteric's body is to retrospectively invest the hysteric with imaginary potential for the sexualisation of the self, which in turn makes it possible for the hysteric to enter the real world of sexual engagements with a new internal set of expectations.

The psychoanalyst, then, is a combined mother and father, a figure who cures the hysteric by using the father's symbolic function to evoke and transform the infant's memory of the mother. When the analyst signals a desire to speak about the patient's body, doing so within a space that has elicited the infant–mother relation, he or she immediately creates a father and a mother who desire one another, and who desire their child's body. If there are reasons why psychoanalysis can itself contribute unwittingly to the endless suffering of the hysteric (in Chapter 12 we will see that there are many such reasons), the very structure of the process itself is curative. All the analyst must do – again and again – is to talk about it whilst the structure acts itself out. The cure is eventually signified by disinterest, as analyst and patient become concerned with other matters.

Notes

1   Throughout this text, unless otherwise stated, when referring to the genital, or the impact of the genital upon the child, I am not referring to the genital stage of psychic integration, nor even to what psychoanalysts term the phallic stage (the era of sexual excitation just prior to the genital stage), but to the differing psychic registrations of genital excitation upon the mind. The differing parts of the body have psychic histories: there is the story of the mouth, the legend of the anus, the tale of the ear, the history of the genital, and so forth.

2   The genital self includes the history of the infant's experience of his or her genital excitations and does not refer only to the genital stage.

3   For a discussion of the concept of the 'unthought known' see my *The Shadow of the Object* (Bollas, 1985).

Chapter 5

Erotising absence

The mother's comings and goings create an absence, which becomes an important form of presence in anyone's life, but the hysteric feels that her absence is driven by an intense withdrawal from her child's sexuality, a rift that presents and re-presents itself as an erotic question between child and mother. It seems an absence saturated by a sexual decathexis of the self that inspires in the child desire-as-yearning. As we shall discuss later, the hysteric absents himself or herself to create a lack in the other, not simply eliciting desire (for the departing hysteric), but instantiating the desire of the other as a form of lack.

Lack[1] would be meaningless without presence and the hysteric also creates forms of presence to play off absence. Sudden abstention from communication is often very arresting. It is not only (as discussed in the last chapter) an invitation to the libidinalisation of internal objects through storytelling in one another's presence: recall from Chapter 3 that Freud linked the 'absences' that typify the hysteric to auto-erotic reveries as he concluded that the 'gap in consciousness' characteristic of the hysterical absence becomes a void which is 'widened in the service of repression', so that it becomes an agency that can 'swallow up every-thing that the repressing agency rejects'. The means of self protection, therefore, are themselves erotised – very subtly so, but it helps in the understanding of the hysteric's abrupt departures. 'Would you tell me what you mean by what you have been saying?' expressed in a lilting and semi-dazed tone of voice may be an auto-erotic spell, the hysteric saturated in the pleasure of innocence.

One aspect of hysterical dissociation derives from the maternal split of the child's erotic being. Whilst ignoring the child's body self as her erotic object, she objectifies before his or her eyes, through performance and narrative, a spectral child whom she engages in highly sensuous ways. It is as if she were reading a book held out in front of her, that is the story of her love of this child, to which she directs the child's attention, riveting him or her to the story through gaze and voice.

Any telling or performing, however, may be at variance with the true state of interrelating, especially with adult hysterics, who seem skilful narrators of their lives, but for whom sexual representation and narrative are strangely at odds with each other. When describing a non-sexual situation they may act in sexually suggestive ways, through gestures and illocutionary acts (Searle 1979: 1), but when addressing sexual life they often do so in an indifferent tone of voice. If the hysteric giggles seductively whilst describing a mundane daily task, it is an invitation to the analyst to invade the patient's inner world with a question. If the question is asked, the hysteric will retreat, showing the analyst what happens if one pursues the desire of the other.

How is one to account for the immanent sexuality of the hysteric? Why, if they are in conflict with genital sexuality, do they so often appear sexual, even when they are refusing it?

We have suggested that the hysteric erotises the work of absence, so that in removing sexuality from psychic and interpersonal realities the sequestration is sexualised. We have added that the body becomes a genitally decentred erotic vehicle, over-sexualising the other erotic zones, often a maternally displaced excitement that the self struggles to contain and also to gratify. How does this evolve?

Again, what the hysteric does is what all children do, although with greater intensity and for compensatory reasons; that is, the hysteric finds in auto-erotism a sensorial release of his or her instinctual life which is gratifying. However, as the scene of the auto-erotic, juxtaposed with the allo-erotic, is in the imaginary, hysterics evolve a somewhat peculiar autosexuality. They imagine themselves the mother's secret object of desire and then, through self-stimulation, erotise this object, which is either narrated back to the mother or performed in her presence. As the mother's sexuality is also auto-erotically based, her narrations and performances express love of the internal object at the expense of the other.

 Mother and child cultivate an alternative erotics based on the pleasures of failed suppression. Ostensibly, the mother refuses to touch the infant's genitals – or does so with ambivalence – but absence of touch suggests its own sexuality. Perhaps, the child wonders, the mother's erotic life is too powerful to be released upon the self. In the absence of such stimulation, however, the child caresses himself or herself, increasing the quantity of sexual mental contents, those not shared with the other. During such self-stimulations the child is momentarily absent from his or her world, caught up in a reverie, evident to others by the child's distracted look. In time he or she will see such a look upon the mother's face – perhaps like the smile of the Mona Lisa – reflecting the pleasure of unseen desires. This look becomes an erotic object shared between the two. At the same time, the body is almost continuously excited by life, on the verge of being overwhelmed by the phantom touch of experience.

Karl Abraham (1913) argued that the ear is an erogenous zone. Sound – we need only think of the mother's cooing – can function as an erotic medium. Lacan (1977) argued that the gaze is also an erotic object, and we may see from the above how the mother's gaze, which touches upon the child at the moment that it confers absented desire, can be hyperinvested with erotic charge. Indeed, in the early moments when two lovers-to-be first meet, it will be by these non-physical erotic means – sight and sound, or gaze and voice – that erotic communication is accomplished. The courtly love tradition stops here and then celebrates absence itself as an erotic fulfilment, elaborated in countless tellings of unrequited love, as with Dante and Beatrice or Petrarch and Laura.

Maternal absence for the hysteric is understood to be an erotic action, a paradoxical moment in which physical touch of the sexual body is either displaced to non-tactile forms of touch – voice and gaze – which suggest that true desire is always absent from self–other realisation, or so disseminated to the other parts of the body as to create a pan-sexuality in constant tension, since no genital binding can be obtained to relieve the body of its sex-ache.

Adult analysands of more florid hysterical mothers can recall how the mother would work herself up into a curious state of self-stimulated erotic intoxication, not suggesting a course toward sexual intercourse with the father, but a narrative– performative ecstasy of its own, leaving the body spent afterwards.

A patient.

> My mother loved going to the movies or reading novels that were love stories. She would come home from a film, or her reading room, full of excitement. If she had just seen Ava Gardner and Rock Hudson in a film she was insistent not only on telling us about the film, but about being Ava Gardner, whom she would act out in our presence. In fact for several days she would *be* Ava Gardner, still talking like her, and insisting that if her life had been different she would have certainly become a great actress. But the compelling thing to all of us was, that although we would tease her and all that, that she was actually caught up in some sort of erotic trance, like someone possessed by a spirit. It was very intense and if we were too mocking in our reply she could go off in a fury telling us we were all ingrates and she did not know why she had anything further to do with us.

There is an interesting collaboration between the mother's and the child's separate auto-erotisms.

As just discussed, through narrative and performance the mother creates the child's double before his or her very eyes, as if saying: 'Look here you are, in my stories about you, and in my performing you in front of yourself.' The child adopts this self as an erotic companion, a specular creature invested by mother and child. This is the object of desire that brings them together. In time, however, this intermediate sex object is taken by the child to be a self extension.

Another patient.

> I can't claim to have known my mother very well and she was not physically very affectionate, although I knew that in her own way she loved me and was obviously intensely interested in me. This was most apparent when she would take me shopping. We would go into clothes stores and there she would dress me up in differing styles and colour combinations as she saw fit. She had this unbelievable intensity during these occasions, plus all kinds of theories about

what sort of outfit to wear and what sort of colour to use at any given time of the year. It was a little spellbinding. So she would dress me up and, get this, she would call me her 'little doll'. The odd thing is that I knew I really in my own self was not her little doll, but looking into the mirror all dressed up at a store, seeing the look of almost total excitement on her face, I thought this little doll me was pretty exciting too. Indeed I elaborated it. I developed my own way of walking and a new style of talking, and certain sorts of precocious hobbies, and it felt as if I were inside some kind of love cult. My mother was in heaven and so in some ways was I and we were both in love with this doll, who was me.

And a third patient.

My mother used to call me her 'little man' and she would say it in a way that was indescribably sexy. It's embarrassing to say it, but early on I can recall getting a genital twinge when she would say it, becoming almost excited. A kind of image of myself would spring to mind when she would say 'little man', and sometimes when she would buy me a new outfit, she would put me in it, then stand back and gaze at me, call me her little man, and then run her hands smartly across my shoulders, straightening my outfit, and then sometimes running her hand down my back in a kind of crisp but lovely way. Other than that, however, she never touched me. Still, I got to say that I sure was pleased that she liked this little man and the image turned me on too.

This double self reflects a type of dissociation common to the hysteric. On the one hand, the true self is sexually suspended, but an intermediate self can be cultivated, based on the auto-erotics of mother and child.

Mother and child then 'marry' through a common renunciation of realised desire, but if the mother is deeply secret and does not suggest her life with her child then, as we shall see, the child may feel frozen by maternal inhibition, rather incarcerated in maternal silence. In psychoanalysis such persons often experience the analyst's silence as just such an incarceration, and the erotic transference demands the substantial materialisation of what is presumed to be the analyst's secret desire.

Masud Khan (1983: 52) maintains that the hysteric attempts to make up for the relative lack of maternal care through a precocious sexual development in which sexual states are exploited in order to make up for deficiencies in the mother's affective and ego support. This leads to a type of grudge in the hysteric with his or her own sexual appeal, as sexuality is exploited for the lack of maternal care. To my way of thinking, the hysteric splits the self, accepting the illusion that the self is in fact a doll-like object which creates an interesting false self – as an invention of desire – that becomes a lure for the other. As we shall see, this predisposes hysterics to be easily misunderstood as offering the self as a sex object, especially when they appear sexy or seductive.

What the hysteric does, then, is to cathect his or her body as an object of unconsciously shared, but nonetheless auto-erotic, interest. He or she attends to the body with a certain kind of auto-erotic care, through which a form of parental intensity is found. It is the hysteric who spends a great deal of time grooming the body. If a woman, she is absorbed with make-up and jewellery, all the while constructing the sex object around her body.

The body self is only meant to be charged by such care; it is not intended to be spent in intercourse with the other. Hysterics do, however, engage in intercourse and the highly complex ways they do so will be discussed later, but they often use sexual encounters as 'banking' events, collecting scenery for auto-erotic life. They may even be sexually promiscuous, but such sexual events charge auto-erotic existence. The self present in intercourse is always the double, the intermediate sex object that stands in for one's desire. There is always an important psychic distance between the hysteric's inner self state and the hysteric's sexual encounters, like a virginal puppet-master manipulating his or her image as a sex object for the other.

A patient puts it succinctly.

> I actually did not stay around with a woman very long. I would see a woman at a party or some place and find her immediately intensely satisfying. I would wonder to myself what she looked like unclothed. And I would really get into seducing her, but no sooner had we fucked than I virtually lost all interest in her. Except that, a few days later, or a week, I would imagine her when masturbating, and that would be fine. After all, it was like having a sexual relation and not the obligations that come with it. And as I have had a lot of women, there are a lot of differing figures I can call upon in my mind whenever I am horny. The sexy me anyway is not who I truly am, but I could get off on appearing to be this dude for the ladies. With 'x' [a girlfriend of some months] I got into the part for quite some time, trying to believe it, but one day it just vanished like waking up from a dream.

Love-making is a mediated sexual encounter occupied by a sexy self. An auto-erotic figure engages the other in intercourse.

A patient.

> I have never been with a man when I was not at the same time vividly imagining him making love to a woman. It is not me he is making love to. It is always a young, adolescent-like woman with small breasts, who is being pinned down – sometimes bound against her will – and it is the first time she has been penetrated. I find this an incredible turn on, and for the most part I am almost completely unaware of the man I am with.

Self-stimulation supplies the hysteric with what he or she needs. Surrender to the other's idiom of love-making is less possible. The other is intended to be a screen for the projection of an internal object, bearing the hidden object of desire. During sexual intercourse hysterics feel removed from the actual sexual gestures of the other, and their partners often complain about this distance. For in a sense, the hysteric, in making love, has found an accomplice in auto-erotics and what seems to be intercourse is masturbation *à deux*.

One patient described her lover's ravenous intercourse as strange. It was too intense, almost an applied manual of technique:

> Rob and I were married for ten years and whenever we made love I always felt that he exploited my body to complete some very private – I have to say it felt pornographic – fuck with me. He was oblivious not only to my sexual tastes, but each time I tried to get into making love with him, he would pin me back, say 'you are going to love this, baby' and he would motor around my body, licking my thighs, biting my shoulder, sucking my toes, like an artist manqué joining the dots on a page to form the prearranged picture. I never had the courage to tell him. He fancied himself a great lover. He read books and books on sex technique, but shit, I felt like I was some rubber mannequin in a sex technique section of the bookstore. All the rest of the day or night he never seemed sexual at all. I never felt that my body 'met' his body. We never lingered. He doesn't know anything about erotic life.

Auto-erotism makes up for a lack (of mother) that we have understood as a lack that is mother, and furthermore a lack that is the desire of mother. As this mother moves back from erotic communication with the body of the child, she suggests, in her abstentions of sensuality and lack in the real, the presence of her inner world which will fulfil itself. Those children who proceed to wed this feature of the mother use auto-erotism as the body of the mother, so in self-stimulation (conducting self–other sexuality only in the secret inner world of fantasy) they do what mother does and become like her. Sexual fantasies which fill the absence of the other bizarrely enough create what feel like false presences – imagined sexual others – removing the sense of lack which constitutes the erotics of the mother and the self. Therefore the sexual scenes of the hysteric must either be dispensed with, re-establishing lack – and creating a serial hysteric – or constantly recurring erotic fantasies must be repeatedly usurped by disappearances that re-establish lack as the route of desire.

Another patient.

Marie was a mother of three and a 'happily married housewife'. She sought analysis because she was disturbed by a lifelong preoccupation. All day long, every day, she imagined that she was accompanied by a movie idol, who shopped with her in the supermarket and admired her choices, who stood by her in the kitchen as she prepared the food and admired her culinary skills, who travelled with her in the car when she collected her children. He would not be present when her husband was in the room and there were other times when he seemed absent and she pined for him. She knew, of course, that he was not really there; so permanently absent he was the presence of absence. She felt her marriage was invalidated by her investment in this lover who – she regretted to say – though never feelable in the bedroom when she slept with her husband, nonetheless took her away from him. Caught up in her imagination she was permanently distracted, unable to make love to her husband in the state of mind that she felt would be essential to deriving true pleasure from him. She was not present to make use of her erotic knowledge.

But what is erotic knowledge?

The mother loves the infant with her whole body: her breasts for feeding, her chest for sleeping on, her lap for sitting, her knee for bouncing, her arms for enfolding, her hands for countless touchings. She suckles, caresses, wrestles, tickles, pokes and pulls the infant in hundreds of acts of physically delivered knowledge every day. If she is a 'good-enough' mother she will translate not only her unconscious fantasies into body communication, she will also unconsciously interpret her infant's gestural requests through her body.

Maternal body knowledge becomes part of the self's own body knowledge and is precursive to the self's own sensuality, which, whilst it initially derives from maternal transformation of the infant's instinctual and bodily needs, subsequently becomes part of the self's expression of bodily being.

As Freud said, this is a love relation. As the mother's intuitive body knowledge forms the base of erotic knowledge, it returns when lovers surrender to one another's bodies. Lovers initiate and receive specific forms of touch, at certain moments, for certain brief periods of time, with certain types of pressure and release, from certain parts of the body, in a moving and changing intensity driving towards mutual orgasm.

Erotic knowledge is the demand of the other's instinct upon the self for work, beginning with the uterus's pressure on the foetus and later the mother's touch. It is what the body knows about maternal erotic craft that insists upon the logic of body pleasure.

It is a sad fact that many hysterics do not know how to take pleasure in this knowledge. Often rather oblivious to it, absorbed in their own auto-erotic universe, they are not easily teased out of themselves. Yet, through psychoanalysis or the sheer good luck of meeting a gifted lover, they can be released from auto-erotic incarcerations into erotic life.

One patient virtually ran into the consulting room to tell me of one such erotic transformation.

> Okay, so I was with X and she is this relatively new woman I have been telling you about, and you know, I was into imagining my favourite woman, when she did this really amazing thing to me. She bit me gently on the back of my neck and climbed on my back. This threw me. It sent a chill up my spine. And then she dipped down and I felt her breasts touch my back and she bit me again, and then . . . it's hard to remember what happened after that. All I know is that I 'lost it' in the best way. My fantasy practically left my body and we

were just into one another. It has never been like that for me with a woman in my life. It was like she was teaching me something and when I sucked her ear she gave a cry of pleasure and well . . . I just can't remember. I think . . . I know it's the first time I've ever actually been made love to and the first time I have made love to anyone else.

Does concentration on the mother as a predisposing influence mean that she will produce hysterical children? Not necessarily.

The 'good-enough' hysteric mother promotes anti-hysteria, a psychic inoculation against infection by her neurosis. She mocks herself, in effect saying: 'For God's sake kids, don't ever be as screwed up as your mum is about her body and sexuality.' She mobilises anti-hysteria, as she burlesques herself: 'If you all want to have a good sexual life, you will have to go elsewhere.' Apparent rejection actually serves her wish to drive her children away from her neurosis.

First a patient. Then a mother who is an hysteric.

The patient had been reluctant to describe his mother in the analysis, because he thought that she would easily be misinterpreted to seem crazier than she was.

My mother was eccentric. She would burst into tears at family gatherings for no obvious reason, now and then she would tear at her clothing and rip part of her outfit, she would literally act out parts of conversations she had heard and so forth; yet, it was such a part of our family life that I never thought about it much. In fact my brothers and sisters and I – I think – not only thought of this as *mother* but as *mother* in a very good way. We all knew that she was screwed up. But it did not have the sort of impact on us that you might imagine, as it seemed full of irony, as if she was poking fun at herself. It was a little like a kind of stand-up comedian, but that goes too far, as she was not – I think – playing herself for laughs, but she was always letting us know that her antics were not to be taken seriously and we were not to get upset.

This patient loved his mother very much, and along with his brothers and sisters, was sent by her to the father for physical affection, as the latter was more embodied and less ambivalent about sexuality.

A mother recalls this aspect of herself. She is in the midst of a session:

I, oh well, I think the *children* were absolutely marvellous. I . . . I . . . I was you know *absolutely awful* to them at times, completely dreadful, a raving banshee . . . but you see . . . 'X' [the eldest son] was my perfect foil as he was so straight and narrow and he would say . . . several times every day . . . 'Mother! Get a grip!' and I would howl with laughter. I needed this in him and you see . . . I played to it . . . because you know . . . God . . . life can be boring . . . and there was fun in all this. Of course I was terribly screwed up, but I let the children know this . . . there was no doubt about it. I could not cut meat, could not bear references to Christianity, hated their new friends for at least

three days before I then completely fell in love with them, and . . . well, you see
. . . they and I knew that I was not to be taken seriously. They would have been
crazy to take me seriously and they were wonderfully sensible children. I was
the closet loony.

Perhaps this points to a form of anti-hysteria, in which the mother mocks herself and
conveys this to the family. So far as I could figure from her accounts of the
children, they went on to have careers and families and were deeply fond of her. As
we shall see in Chapter 11, when discussing the malignant hysteric, the 'good-
enough' hysterical mother finds a way to break the child's attachment to her
neurosis by becoming slightly mad, in small and ironically loving doses, so that as
the children move into their oedipal period they are no longer looking to the
mother for a kind of sexual confirmation. Its absence, however, does not translate
into an hysterical attack on sexuality itself – at least, it does not inevitably follow
– because the mother has cancelled herself out as the arbiter of erotism.

This mother encourages the child to seek sexual destiny with another type of sex
object, one with a mentality receptive to erotic needs. A part of any self's idiom –
which I see as the peculiar aesthetic of form true to our character – is the drive to
articulate and develop this aesthetics of being, our destiny drive, as it were. The
aim of such a drive is to present and re-present one's idiom, accomplished in part
by selecting and using objects through which to develop. Understood as part of the
life instinct, the destiny drive is the urge to use objects in order to come into being
and relating expressive of one's true self, and this is the primary impetus behind
the allo-erotic choice. By desiring the other – and objects in the world – the self
finds a complex vocabulary of objects through which to speak the self, but auto-
erotism is a fundamentally different drive, more like the work of the death instinct
– in which objects are selected in order to extinguish desire. At best, the hysteric's
auto-erotism is the past's desire of itself and the colonised object world serves the
self's sexual fate, rendering the hysteric a passive recollector rather than an active
seeker. The mother's anti-hysteria breaks the spell not only of past object choices,
but of the past as object of desire. In its place is the future, there to fulfil the self's
destiny through the fortunes of chance arrivals of objects found to be desirable.
Whereas the hysteric eroticises a past that visits the self in fateful reveries, the non-
hysteric eroticises the future as he or she continues to seek the object to fulfil the
desire.

The death-drive hysteric dissociates the self from erotic relatedness, finding in
maternal absence the preferred space for the construction of a maternal erotic
object sought after only in auto-erotic states. The aim of erotic engagement is to
extinguish the instincts, reducing levels of excitation. The mother, perhaps more
alive-in-herself than the child, is continuously present as an excitational force, so
the child is forced to put her in a distant place.

The death-drive hysteric exploits maternal ambivalence and uses it in a vengeful
way, withdrawing the self from the parents in order to punish them through a
decathexis meant to leave them out in the cold. There is an intense envy of the

primal scene as the imagined place of true love (and maternal cathexis) that the hysteric now hates by removal. The death-drive hysteric may seduce the other's desire in order to take revenge on the primal scene by declining intercourse at the last moment, or in its aftermath becoming enraged and vengeful toward the lover. The sexual scene is always the mother's and father's place and the death-drive hysteric feels that his or her own participations are concessions to parental authorship. Unlike the life-drive hysteric, who seeks the mother's love and strives to realise her desire, the death-drive hysteric kills off maternal love and systematically takes revenge on the other's expectations.

When considering maternal influence on any self's character perhaps it is best to keep in mind that we all have borderline, schizoid, hysteric (etc.) structures latent to our personality. A mother's frame of mind with any one of her infants may sponsor an intensification of one of the character structures. In a family of five children, for example, a mother may evoke borderline fusion with one infant but schizoid detachment with another, or an hysteric response from yet another. Finally, it is the child's ego that will elect its own strategy, moving toward one or another of the character structures that it determines is best for the unconscious needs of the self.

Enough about the mother and her infant. What about the father?

Note

1   'Lack' is a term used by Lacan in a highly specific way. Although aspects of his theory bear on my own use of the term, to avoid confusion the reader should not take my use to be an accurate application of Lacan's idea.

Chapter 6

Functions of the father

The ordinary essential predisposition towards the father is suggested in the first place by the mother, who refers to all his functions: as a figure in the family imaginary, as the upholder of the law held in his name, and as the out-of-sight other ready to arrive from the real. Not only will she talk about this daddy, she will also indicate her own loving feelings towards him. So from the very beginning he will be a vital third object referred to many times over, preparing the infant for his second coming, which lies ahead in the oedipal period.

In the good life, the father may participate in the early childhood of his daughter or son. Although his presence is not equivalent to any of the above functions – symbolic, imaginary, real – it is nonetheless an important feature in the child's experience of those functions. We might think of this father as transitional, somewhere between the work of mothering in the maternal order and the work of fathering in the paternal order.

If so, he joins the mother in her evolution from bearer of the maternal order to co-leader of the paternal order. Forms of being and relating, these orders operate according to different psychic functions associated with the name of the mother or the father. Actual mothers and fathers work in both orders.

Before proceeding, however, let us think further about what is meant by the maternal and paternal orders. When psychoanalysis refers to the internal mother or the internal father it includes imagoes of the self's mother and father, it assumes aspects of the self's idiom projected into these internal objects, and finally it refers to inner psychic structures. There is a structure in the name of the mother and a structure in the name of the father. These structures, in turn, are composed of their functions. When referring to the separate set of functions, we may now refer to the maternal and paternal orders, especially if we intend to emphasise the functional difference between the two. The psyche is not unisexual, but bisexual, and a self will be utilising separate but equal sets of functions. In referring to the internal mother or the maternal order we include the psychic functions of reception, gestation, delivery and holding, as well as forms of communication based on non-verbal means. In referring to the internal father or the paternal order, we include the functions of penetration, insemination, guardianship, encountering, law-making and enforcement, and when specifying this type of communication we refer to the Mosaic function.

Freud's theory of the unconscious recognises the difference between these two structures. The primary repressed unconscious is composed of 'thing presentations', inner organisations derived from accumulated experiences – visual, somatic, kinaesthetic, acoustic – of the object world. The self is receiving the objects of its world before it can think this in words and this pre-verbal processing of life occurs under the auspices and the intuitive direction of the mother whose own body has held the infant inside her and who for many months has come to know her infant through her soma, her affects and her imaginings: a form of knowing and communicating that both mother and child inherit and use in the first months of life. She may tell the father about the infant, but he is always on the outside. What might seem unfortunate for him – as a distinct outsider – is vital to the survival and eventual psychic prosperity of the mother–infant couple, as pregnancy and early childcare are deep indwellings when both mother and infant are vulnerable to threats from the outside. Protecting this space, thinking of its needs in relation to reality, and if necessary challenging reality to protect the couple, is an archaic function of the father. As the infant becoming a child will discover over time, there are many parts of a life that all along are outside the infant–mother relation. The words mother used to put the baby's body into song were not invented by her, but derived from the complex structure of language, which follows grammatical rules watched over by, amongst others, the custodians of language in the theological and academic worlds – very far away from the infant's experience of reality.

Being composed of thing presentations in the first place means that the primary repressed unconscious is full of unthought-known forms of knowledge waiting for developed forms of thinking to evolve, so that part of what is known is eventually available for representation in speech, imagination, affect or enactment. Freud's theory of the unconscious is almost exclusively focused on the secondary repressed unconscious, when the self can begin to think its thoughts in language and can repress ideas it finds objectionable – inevitably, according to Freud, ideas that are driven by the pre-verbal infant, whose instinctual requirements force ideas on any self from the body. The inner 'no' and censorship in the child directed at such contents increasingly finds in the father's presence an organised structure of 'no's, of laws and consequences to which the self must adapt if it is to survive. Thus banishing ideas is associated with the function of banishment – of exiling the unwanted, an archaic structure of the father in the unconscious life of the self. In *Oedipus Rex* it is Laius, not Jocasta, who authorises the banishment of Oedipus, who returns to bed his mother only after he has killed the father.

When referring to the maternal and paternal orders, then, we also simultaneously refer to the two dimensions of the unconscious: the work of the primary repressed unconscious and the work of the secondary repressed unconscious. The primary repressed unconscious I take to function according to the maternal order, whose basic 'law', if we like, is one of *reception*. The secondary repressed unconscious I take to function according to the paternal order and follows the law of *repression*. To invite, to repel. Yes, no. Binary opposition. In the inner world, the internal mother and the internal father have essential intercourse every day. Indeed, so too in Freud's theory itself, as thing presentations can only become available to consciousness by attaching themselves to words, so the inner mother world and the inner father world constantly link and create third objects that shall be born of this coupling.

The hysteric tries to make an alliance with this couple only on the grounds of a false self that mandates it to go forward as a model citizen, as an enticing love object. The hysteric seeks to remain in the impressionistic envelope of the maternal order: in affectionalist, visual and acoustic embrace. The laws of the awaiting outside world strike the hysteric as a violent rupture of this envelope. The hysteric's solution is to do whatever can be done to undermine the lucidity of the paternal law by creating confusions, seeking to bring out in the mind of the self and its others mother-envelopes, composed of affect states operating to deny access to the father. At very best, the hysteric will daydream reality, even implementing the daydream to significant lasting effect, but this applied psychic literature is a skilful manipulation of reality according to the magic realism of the inner envelope. As Freud (and later Winnicott) indicated, it is in art and cultural creation that the self ordinarily does this, nourishing the two sides of the self's investments: the world of the deep unconscious – wordless always – and the world of sparkling objects and linguistic cover.

So, to return to the hysteric's journey. When the mother conveys desire for her child's bodily being, joined with the father's desire of the mother, it reads as follows: 'Mother desires my body. As father desires mother, he desires her desire and therefore he too desires me.'

With the child moving towards an hysteria there are problems. First, the mother does not include the father as a desired third object. There may be situational reasons for this, such as the father abandoning mother and child, which results in the mother's elimination of him from her discourse, turning him into a failing third object. Or, if the mother is characterologically an hysteric, then she would be likely to convey two differing fathers: an ideal object that would be magical and unreal, and an ambivalently regarded real object that would be persecutory. She might think of him as sexually dangerous or physically repulsive.

Second, the actual father may be disturbed, discrediting his functions. If the mother's ambivalence is severe, then it may marry the father's self cancellations, leaving the child uncertain how to use a combined mother and father, or how to integrate the functions that operate in the maternal and paternal orders. This disturbance can be quite severe and, as we shall find in our discussion of malignant hysteria (Chapter 11), these are likely to be parents who refuse their orders and then act out in front of the children. For the moment, however, we will consider the less disturbed hysteric.

The hysteric temporarily solves the problem of ambivalence by using the false self to stand in place of inner convictions. This feels self-sacrificial, as the child has had to suspend inner psychic reality for outward appearances, and when this operates in relation to the father, the child makes the following statement: 'I give up my true desires and comply with what is expected of me by giving you what you want.' The child then constructs a theory of paternal narcissism, which might read as follows: 'You who dominate mother and me demand that we accede to your image, which we do. We only do so because of your power. We cannot overpower you. I shall accept your laws only in order to grow strong enough so that one day I may remove you.' As this father partly stands for reality, let us now read this as an address to reality: 'Reality. Mother and I were fine until you came along and disrupted us. I hate you, reality, but I must accept that I cannot overpower you. I shall adapt to you. But one day, when I am grown up, I shall overpower you, renounce you, and return to mother.' The hysteric is the figure who seeks success in order to renounce it, who throws off work and relations in mid-life to seek a different existence. All along he or she has adapted in order to return to an imagined ideal world.

A patient captures something of this state of mind as he describes a part of his life:

> So anyway, I am slogging away at work as usual, putting in the nine to five, and I hate my job. The place [a university] is a factory, just churning out one useless academic after the next. I have been working all my life, since I was 20. I've never had a break and to be frank I'm fed up with it. Why should I have to keep struggling like this? And it sucks to have to keep sending most of my money to [his former wife] who just bleeds me dry. Who needs this shit? Nah . . . I'm tired, I'm fed up, I have been struggling all my life and it's time I thought of myself instead of others. What I need is to get out of the rat race, to get the fuck out of the city, and back to [he names an island off the Northwest American coast] where I can just hang out and recover from the shitheads of this world. I should not have to go on like I've been doing . . .

This patient had always felt his father was critical and disapproving of him, and he has much the same feeling towards his colleagues and seniors at the university. By extension, the city, the world, even life itself, feels like it has been a demanding intrusion into what could have been – and should be in the future – a more idyllic existence. As the analysis proceeded, he realised that however upsetting his actual father's bad behaviours had been, these were memorable because he was attacking the internal father as well, a father as tutor of delayed gratification, self-sacrifice, obligation and performance. By attacking the father, he had simultaneously assaulted reality, thereby undermining his own creativity and productivity.

The hysteric experiences the father as a figure whose power grows in inverse ratio to what the child loses. What is lost is the illusion of singular union with the mother, and by the time the child enters the oedipal stage, part of which is the era of full recognition of the father's status, the hysteric is already feeling that his or her power has been displaced by the father. This is an interesting twist to the classic story of Oedipus. In Sopholces's drama, Laius gets rid of his son because it has been prophesied that the son will kill him, and in the course of the play the child kills his father without knowing who he is. In fact, another legend of a child's Oedipus conflict would have to reverse this plot. The son would already be king, unaware that the father would one day 'kill' him by revealing that he sleeps with the mother, a crossroads in the child's life that unseats him from the throne. In psycho-development we are all 'mother-fuckers', born from the mother's womb to suckle her breasts, engaged in a long period of mutual love-making with her. Then this figure whom we dimly perceived – and have sent packing to another place – returns to kill us without knowing who we are!

At the same time, however, the 'return of the father' proves to be a vital and essential 'killing' of the self, as it is through matriculation into the paternal order that the child separates from the infant self and from the mother of that self. Indeed, father-the-obstacle[1] proves vital to the child's negotiation with all future difficulties, and boys and girls seek conflict with this otherwise unwanted figure, unconsciously knowing that in doing so they are serving their own futures.

The hysteric recognises this. He or she knows that going forward is essential in order to survive, but equally that it is by now part of the pledge of precocity – of being a good boy or a good girl – and that to 'adopt' the father is also essential. This is accomplished by manic identifications with the adult sides of the mother and the father, realised in these children, who become perfect little women or perfect little men. The skill developed in discovering and enacting maternal desire works on their behalf as they now provide the father (i.e. reality) what he desires. But fulfilling the father's desire is not equivalent to engaging the father-as-obstacle. Identifying with his desire strangely incarcerates the child in the maternal order, declining those trials and tribulations that await the child who truly takes on the father's law and all that it suggests.

One function of the castration complex is to mobilise an anxiety in relation to the father, who will embody the impingement of the real upon any self's unconditional relation to the mother. This anxiety is, then, ultimately related to those castrations performed by reality, such as the recognition of parental sexuality, the birth of a sibling, the discovery of other families, the demands of school, the arbitrary selections of the peer group, and so forth. Battling the father is akin to engaging reality. What does the hysteric do with this anxiety?

In a sense, the good girl and the good boy become Barbie children, who have suspended the true self in order to realise what they imagine to be parental desire. That these children *are* unusually good means that they are highly prized objects in contemporary Western culture. This may be more evident with the good girl who sets herself up as teacher's helper and who appears exceptionally mature, deleting from her behaviour both sexual curiosity and aggressive elaborations, all the while concerned to be as grown up as the adults around her. One can often discern the strain in these children, from the boy who seeks to be 'macho' as the little man – and may be outstanding in sports, academic study and community relations – and the coquettish little woman who is intelligent, charming and feminine. Each of these children strains to evolve a false self, constructed on precocious manic identifications with the adult world, leaving in a corner of the self an unprocessed infantile being that has not been taken along on this journey. Further, as this strain is also informed by castration anxiety, there is a fear in these children, and later as adults, that something awful is going to intervene in their lives to destroy all their assumptions and accomplishments.

Identification with the father's desire accomplished through false-self precocities evades engagement with the father, which in some respects is a castration of the father's function. These boys and girls, whilst appearing charming, are in fact deferring a refusal of the father until later in life – a defiance that may take a violent turn, just as these false identifications with the father's desire have also been a form of defiance.

This is a complicated matter. On the one hand, the 5- or 6-year-old child appears very grown up in a way and could continue thus through adolescence and into adult life proper. On the other hand, this development is driven by certain anxieties and, with the true self suspended, it is a fragile kind of progress. Indeed, and at what point does the common hysteric trait of sustaining the child self – and refusing the adult self – manifest itself? How can we reconcile this apparent contradiction, between the child who appears to be adult and the adult who will live as a child?

In fact, the contradiction has existed from the very moment that the child assumed a false identity. For this *is* a performance: the good boy and the good girl are unreal manifestations of the internal world, even if they are celebrated by society. This little man and this little woman have leapfrogged into adulthood in such a way as to transcend sexuality in their childhoods.

How can this be? If they have jumped into adult apparitions, would this not mean they have done exactly the opposite, that they have therefore rushed into the sexual? It would appear so, but by overtly expressing sexuality as performance – in the coquettish little girl or the macho little boy – the child presents, rather than experiences, sexuality. In adult life, these men and women may sustain the paradox of this accomplishment, appearing quite seductive and sexual, but when called upon by a lover to sustain sexuality, turning away from it and seeking to return to seductive presentations as an alternative to encountering sexuality.

Precocious identification with the imagery of adult life eliminates the child's identification with the name of the father and constitutes an ambivalent attitude towards the paternal order. Indeed, the child will often unconsciously castrate the father's phallus by transforming the father's function into a 'teddy daddy', a figure meant to be a cuddly object that serves to marginalise both the phallus and the father's tougher function as the arbiter of reality. By idealising this father, the hysteric cancels out sexuality and the father proceeds as a desexualised object.

The hysteric's idealisation of the father is very common, but, as in the idealisation of the mother, the aim is to desexualise the object. The ideal (the desexualised father) is installed as the prototype of the good man, one who – it is unconsciously assumed – has accepted his castration as the law-giver. The hysteric imagines him to be the parent who now authorises the hysteric's permanent status as an ideal child. The most common example of this formation is the hysteric woman who idealises her father, to whom no man can compare. Being 'daddy's girl' is a lawful exemption from the ordinary, the self a princess in a fairy-tale existence. This father has a throne in the permanent structure of the self's daydream, an *imaginary* symbolic figure. So, although this is the self's father, in fact, he is a stand-in for the structure of the mother, the self now sustained in a new family, an ideal world never to be disrupted by the defining maturational force of sexual recognitions.

However, as acceptance of the paternal order is essential to authorised and invigorated participation in culture and society, the desexualised father is a crippled function in the self. What has been gained in the idealisation of the father has been lost in the denial of the phallus, which disempowers the self. This conflict is to varying extents comprehended by hysterics. They are in conflict with two very different notions of personal evolution. They know that if they are fully to enter the paternal order then they must accept reality, psycho-development and certain losses of the mother. To refuse this path would be to reconstitute the self through life in the maternal order. Thus, hysterics are stuck in a kind of limbo, usually attempting to do both, but winding up in a kind of psychic stalemate.

A patient.

> Basically I am two people. At work I am very responsible and mature and people think highly of me. When I walk out of the house and ride on the train to work I am genuinely looking forward to my day and to the work that I must do. I like the way I look, that is the way I dress, and much of the time I take it to be really me, although I am somewhere always sort of watching myself from some admiring distance, so it is also in a way an act. But it is an act which is okay with me. I suppose that is the case, because when I cross the front door of my home, I collapse into a total child. I change into my running gear, and to the annoyance much of the time of my lover, I speak in baby talk. I have pet names for everything and I am a very little boy. When my partner complains about the comparative absence of our sex life I tell her I don't like sex: in a sort of mocking and petulant way. When we do make love I am surprised to enjoy it, but afterwards I run from her body, which quite frankly I find rather off-putting. But I am grateful for my dick in a way, as when it – I call it Tommy – when Tommy wants to do it, well that's okay with me, and I kind of go along for the ride.

This patient, in his early thirties, was upset by the split in his life and by the degree of his childlike behaviour at home. He knew it was a drain on his partner, but he could also feel the regressive pull within himself; he too felt depleted by it. On the other hand, he loved the comfy world he had created out of his pet names and his baby talk, and he greatly enjoyed being a small child comforted in a kind of 'mummy world'. He knew that this drew him away from the mentality he entered when he went to work and he could see how the two dispositions were at odds with one another. In fact, he was struck by sudden anxiety attacks, which on further analysis proved to be occasioned by his shifts from one frame of mind to the other, much of which amounted in any one moment to an attack on the other order. At home he was in unconscious opposition to the paternal order, at work in opposition to the maternal order, and whenever he went from one world into the next his anxiety registered the fear of being mutilated by the offended order.

Hysterics are usually able to describe this conflict between the child and the adult self. They can also recall thinking as children about the problems of growing up, and they also remember their aversion to sexuality. If they have used the manic side of their false-self development – that precocity which allows them magically to materialise as young adults at 5 – in adult life to reach another person sexually, they also know that this euphoric moment is short-lived and that revulsion with the other's body – especially the genitalia – is forthcoming. If they take comfort in the power of the instincts to anaesthetise the self against its psychic revulsions through its intoxicating drive, they know that after orgasm the anaesthesia will wear off and they will be confronted with the real body of the other.

Another patient.

> Well quite frankly I just never understood what the hell always happened to me. It didn't matter what woman I was with. When I was excited and had an erection their bodies were almost perfect, although I know that I didn't quite see their bodies as I had an image of them more in my mind than anything else. But still I imagined a very desirable object. But no sooner had I come and rolled off them, then when I looked at them, what I saw was 'flesh', by which I mean something rather unappealing. And I never wanted to see the cunt. If I did it always sent shivers up my spine. It always looked like some slimy oyster, and I could hardly believe I had ever wanted to fuck that.

Not surprisingly, hysterics are not at all sure they actually want to marry when it comes right down to it. When people bolt from the wedding day, usually it is the hysteric taking flight from the reality of imminent commitment to sexual life with an other and to body-to-body co-existence. But throughout life, hysterics have always felt themselves to be amidst difficult choices: to be with mother or with father; to be a child or to assent to becoming an adult; to be alone and auto-erotic or to be with the other and allo-erotic. Interestingly, they find compensation in this engagement with the father and his order through an intriguing privileging of choice. They find in the idea of choice, which is in many respects a dilemma, the basis of a strength. That is to say, they emphasise that the choice, or the choosing, is to be one's own special privilege. An example will help clarify this rather elusive point.

At a dinner party there were about fifteen people engaged in convivial dialogue and enjoying one another's company. One woman seemed somewhat ill at ease, however, frowning as others conversed. As the dinner was ending the host asked if everyone would like to go for a short walk to the ice-cream store where they could buy cones and then return for coffee. Everyone assented spontaneously except for the woman described. She did not decline, though. Instead, she paused, long enough for most of the people present to look her way to see what she thought.

Her reply was interesting. She said: 'I could do that.' By this she did not mean that as she could do it she therefore would do it; rather, the way she put it, she meant that as it was something within her capability it was therefore fair enough for her to think about it. A friend nudged her a bit and said, 'Ah come on, you'll like it', to which she replied, 'But I have a choice in this and I haven't decided.' Another person said, 'Ah, she is just thinking about it, so let's give her time', during which the woman looked pensive, drawn into herself for a moment. Then she smiled wanly and said, 'Okay I will come.' The effect on the group was also interesting. Rather than this being an occasion for celebration, it rather took the wind out of the group's sails, and a simple stroll around the block now seemed to be a less pleasant prospect.

It seems to me that what this person did was to privilege her choice over the two options – to stay or to go – and she enacted something that I realised when this incident was first described to me was an important feature of hysterical patients, as, in a manner every bit as subtle, they find a way to become special through the dilemma they face. If it is something of an admirable compromise between two opposing options, it is also, no doubt, frustrating for those who must live with such people as companions.

The woman at the dinner party clearly isolated herself and in a way that would appear schizoid, as her relation to her internal objects openly displaced her relation to actual others who were forced to watch her mull things over with *them* before coming to a decision. But isolation of the self is the alternative route to the precocity described above, as the hysteric may also seek an ascetic solution to the marring effects of sexuality. By denying the body its sexual fulfilments, the ascetic hysteric testifies to the transcendence of sexuality. If the child is unable to marry the mother who refuses her own sexuality, then asceticism also declines all object relating in the interests of self-sacrifice. Indeed, the history of hysteria is as replete with the ascetic hysteric who does without his or her sexuality as it is occupied with the flirt who ornamentalises the instinct by wearing its features as a lure, only to decline its actuality in the end.

Death-drive hysteria takes the ascetic route, attacking the self's sexuality in order to oblate maternal desire (if it existed) and parental sexuality. Later, when discussing the anorectic, we shall see how death-drive hysteria removes self from its body in order to assault the expectations of the parental world.

We have, then, two fundamentally different hysteric solutions to the anguish of sexuality: the ascetic and the precocious. Ascetic hysteria derives its passion from maternal decathexis of the body and uses anti-libido as its force. It is death-drive hysteria. As we have seen in Petrarchan love, it is the absence of the object which becomes the source of the self's passion, one that is inevitably masochistic, yet out of what is not physically available comes love of the other as a soul. This is a romance with the death drive and is the passion that leads hysterics to kill themselves.

Precocious hysteria is a manifestation of the life drive, as the hysteric who follows this route cathects the mother's overcompensation for her psychic decathexis of the infant's sexuality. It uses her displaced erotism (recall that this mother sexualises the non-genital surfaces of the infant's body) and combines this with her verbal and theatrical portrayal of their love relation to move the self into the world of adult sexuality with the passionate energy of a type of false self.

But both sides – the precocious adoption of the sexual and the ascetic refusal of it – co-exist in the hysteric, and whilst the one solution may predominate throughout life, it does not mean that its opposite has disappeared altogether. Indeed, promiscuous hysterics may suddenly – and forever – become sexless, whilst ascetic hysterics may suddenly burst into apparent sexiness.

Death-drive hysteria requires further qualifications on our emphasis of the mother's role as a predisposing feature to hysteria. It may be enough for the death-drive hysteric to find in maternal cathexis of the father an enviable flow of libido, which is then interpreted as being derived from maternal decathexis of the self. Add to this the ordinary subsequent events of life, such as the child's castration complex, Oedipus complex, the birth of other siblings, the maturational processes' insistence on itself, and the death-drive hysteric may have had enough of life by the age of 6. The child's silent withdrawal from participation in family, school and community life would seem to the death-drive hysteric a tempting path, as it would be paved with the broken hearts of a small village of people who have tried to dissuade this person from self-destructive behaviour.

The death-drive hysteric's attack on life partly owes its power to the hatred of the body and its sexual needs. St Francis of Assisi, for example, was an adored, spoiled and ribald child. Doted upon by both parents, his character was subsequently muted by a year of imprisonment during the Assisi and Perugia war of 1202 and by a journey in 1205 to fight in the south of Italy, where he probably hoped to establish himself as a hero. No sooner had he departed on his dangerous ordeal – the family and village celebrations fresh in his mind – than he suffered what is likely to have been a failure of courage and returned to Assisi. He claims to have seen a vision in Spoleto, but his parents and friends were disappointed, and then bewildered, by the subsequent abandonment of his appearance. He embraced poverty, hung out with lepers, and began to restore churches. His outraged father demanded he be tried in public in the village square, and at the conclusion Francis disrobed himself – standing naked before his father and fellow citizens – and broke off all affiliations with his family. From this point forward he became a true ascetic and formed his order.

In her fascinating account of his life and his psychology, Nitza Yarom (1992) argues that Francis resolved his conflict with his father by identifying with Jesus and becoming his son, finding that 'the new father–son relationship was clear of ambivalence' (p. 52). Francis was also able to flourish, Yarom argues, through his 'killing' of the father, which enabled him to go on to demonstrate his capabilities as a merchant, fighter and loving brother.

We may see in Francis's asceticism a violent refusal of his sexuality and of the father with whom it is associated. By repudiating the actual father, Francis can join the spiritual father, who is in any event an adored object of his culture. This does indeed offer to the hysteric a certain triumph of sorts, as this 'other' father exists in the imaginations of men and women and is known through different forms of representation, especially scripture and the fine arts. By ascending to the spiritual world, the ascetic hysteric unconsciously returns to the world of the mother and her infant, which is unconsciously asserted in the tendency to privilege Mary with Jesus. Yarom points out that 'in general, in the lives of the medieval saints, it was the mother who supported their new vocation, whilst the father opposed it' (p. 54), something which was also true of Francis's mother. It is of interest, therefore, that Christianity offers an hysterical solution to the problems posed by the sexual father. The story of Jesus, the separation of the sexes in the Catholic clergy and the renunciation of sexuality, the denigration of carnal requirements and the privileging of spiritual virtues, and the celebration of one's departure from earth to a joyful merger with spiritual beings in a better world – these teachings form a conduit for hysterical flight from the violation upon the self of sexuality.

Francis obviously tried to fulfil himself as a conventional man, but failed. Faced with his own disappointment in his character and humiliated by an outraged father, he renounced his earthly father and, in the name of the mother, invoked the privilege of a higher relation.

More commonly, the juxtaposition of these two divergent solutions to sexuality – transcendence by denial, transcendence by false identification – lends the hysteric's presence an often bizarre quality.

A clinical example.

A male patient attended sessions in tight jeans and tight shirts and spoke in a flirtatious manner, caressing the spaces above his body with both hands acting like sexual puppets. When it came to speaking about his sexuality, however, his hands fell to his sides, his body movements stopped, and he adopted a childlike voice that spoke of such matters as if they were dirty.

A female patient attended sessions in entirely different outfits and was often exceedingly flirtatious and sexy. In such hours she was talkative and engaging and sought to be quite entertaining. In other sessions she appeared in dark clothing, was silent most of the time, and totally disengaged. This split in her being is of course quite common to the hysteric's self presentations, as we shall discuss later, and the genesis of what the hysteric may choose to present as a multiple personality disorder, that is, if he or she can find a clinician for whom this is an object of desire.

Aside from this presentation of two rather different selves, hysterics commonly float possible selves like trial balloons. Like the child who emerges from a cinema acting out one of the characters, the hysteric emerges from readings or social engagements acting out aspects of a character he or she has seen or imagined. Each of these imagined selves is rather like a *past* past self floating in future time, in ongoing experimentation with the arts and crafts of ontology.

As discussed in the previous chapter, the non-hysteric assimilates the adult world, deferring genital sexuality until some future time, but the hysteric identifies with any object from the past, which it carries by identification into its future.

More than any of the other characters of psychoanalysis, the hysteric is deeply ambivalent about growing up. Being a charming girl or boy, a beguiling man or woman, seems compromise enough; it keeps the child self positioned against the adult prospects. Even though these people often go on to achieve a great deal in life, there is a secret bitterness towards the terms of this choice. There is a nagging feeling that in entering the paternal order – even as child actors – they have betrayed their claim on the mother. As the self pushes forward into its new forms, the hysteric begrudges the father his insensitive demand, but castration anxiety is considerable, because the father has been unconsciously attacked, and the hysteric always feels that his or her adult accomplishments will be dashed to bits by a stroke of fate. Such an unconscious anxiety is often anticipated, and in an ironic effort at mastery, managed through dramatic – and usually self-destructive – changes of career, or partner, or family, the hysteric brings about catastrophe on his or her head. Adding to the paradox of this compromise – i.e. self castration as pre-emptive of castration by the other – is its evocation of the very anxieties it seeks to annul, since this effort to triumph over the father by co-opting his function only adds to the unconscious fear that the father has now been attacked once again and one's status is not secure.

Because the hysteric only makes partial use of the father, he or she is aware of losing out: he or she could have had a more robust engagement with this figure and with social reality. Herein lies a type of sadness – over what is lost – and the structure of hysterical melancholy: the hysteric has lost the true self's participation in existence. Instead, the understudy has taken over the role of the self and brilliantly portrayed its participation in social reality; but engaging with reality and playing at it are quite different. The pain of falsification is increased as the hysteric observes other people clearly engaging in their work and participating in society. The normal other carries part of the hysteric's true self, imagined in the other through projective identification. This second loss dynamically feeds the melancholic structure, made worse by a type of envy peculiar to the hysteric: envy of the other's maturity. As always, envy diminishes the self just as it over-empowers the other, and the hysteric's lot is to feel further infantilised by the cycle of projective identification of the true self and envy of the other for its increased maturational pleasures. The hysteric seeks compensation in maturation-daydreamed, leaping ahead of others not through actual accomplishments, but through imagined ones. The imaginary order is meant to compete with and usurp the symbolic order; daydreaming is meant to triumph over invigorated engagements with social reality, biasing the hysteric to take continual refuge in a system of thought that favours the imagining of self and reality over participations of self in reality.

The effort to act in the name of the mother weakens the hysteric's ego and further diminishes the self's ability to engage reality. Matters are made worse if the father himself is hysteric. How does the hysteric father influence his child's development?

First, a description of a male hysteric; then, his fathering in his own words.

He is a 35-year-old businessman who is very successful in his field, where he is regarded as a somewhat imposing and fearsome figure. In analysis it became clear that this presentation was rather carefully orchestrated and based on his imitation of previous bosses and his readings on leadership. For example, he read in one book that the most effective way to assume power in a new position was to sack several people and thus assert authority, which he did, and indeed it gave him five years' clear run as the manager of a medium-sized company.

When he crossed the threshold from work to home, however, no sooner was he ripping the tie from his neck than he was also dissembling his character to that of a small, impish, often annoying, and sometimes charming little boy. His wife seemed the steady figure in the family who more or less looked after all the children's needs and who seemed prepared to look after her husband when he joined the fray as an early adolescent presence.

Early on in the analysis he talked about how he joined the children in playing all sorts of games, but it became clear that these games were less structured and more like known forms of mayhem, such as a disorganised game of football, or an impromptu game of charades. They were impulsive, often taking place at the wrong time of day – such as just before dinner or bedtime – and he put the children into an 'hysterical' state of mind, as he described it. He systematically declined to help the children with anything that would facilitate their maturation, such as homework, or acquiring a real skill, or experiencing cultural objects, such as films, plays, exhibitions, or the like. He complained that he was 'too tired' or that such enterprises were 'too depressing' as they reminded him of the world of his work, which preoccupied him, he argued, too much as it was.

For the most part the children found him amusing. He clowned a lot. At home he had a high piercing giggle that was infectious. He spoke in cartoon voices, acting out roles that he had established over the years in the home.

It was clear that his wife loved him. He was talented, complex, vulnerable and, in his own way, caring, and I think she was devoted to looking after him, not at all unlike she was with her children. Their relation was intermittently sexual and the patient made it quite clear that he did not really like making love very much. He distinguished between making love and intercourse and said that he preferred to just 'jump' his wife when the mood struck and to move straight to intercourse. The sight of her might suddenly stimulate him – especially if she was wearing a particular dress – or he might be having an erotic fantasy. He did not want to make love (by which he meant anything like foreplay) as he found that looking at her actual body, especially her genitals, was a deterrent and he would lose his erection. He also did not like the sight of his own penis, which he found embarrassing, and indeed always had done – immediate penetration was a way of putting it out of sight.

Of his own fathering, here is what he said one session, after he had discussed his children's being somewhat removed from him during their adolescence. This comment is from the fourth year of analysis, and he is depressed thinking about his own hysteria as a father.

> I think I was a good father, in some ways, but in others not so. I did not want to be a real father: that is, someone who . . . well I didn't know what at the time. I did not want to take authority and I left everything up to 'X' [his wife] as she was more matter-of-fact than I was. I feel sorry in different ways for the children. I failed with my son to give him a proper model of a father and I can see where his own acting out follows mine a bit, as I know I was actually 'attacking' my function of being a father by remaining a boy at home. That was not good for him. And with my daughter, I wanted her love and her affection, which she gave me, but when she was seeking out my 'sexual' confirmation of herself as a sexual being, I know that I acted as if I did not know what she was on about. I never complimented her and never bought her anything for her body and I know that she wanted something 'bought by Daddy' to wear as a kind of emblem of my desire. I just opted out . . .

Perhaps this vignette captures elements of the hysterical father. This would be a man who, as we see, declines to fulfil the functions of the father, but instead joins the children in acting out anti-authoritarian positions. This may have many consequences, not least the failure to validate the child's search for 'sexual licensure': in the case of the daughter, her wishes – amongst others – to wear an object purchased by the father (in the exchange economy of kinship systems that move sex objects out of the house and into other homes); and in the case of the son, to have equivalent licences issued through paternal handings-down.

The male hysteric's refusal to occupy the position of the father, and to represent the father's desire of his wife, amounts to an attack on important psychic structures that are of potential use to the children. Adam Limentani (1989) has offered a portrait of a kind of man, whom he terms 'vagina man', which Juliet Mitchell (1997) argues is a paradigm for a different kind of father operating in juxtaposition to the father of the castration complex envisioned by Freud. Mitchell wonders if we can continue to consider the Freudian father as a model of the nuclear other in the family constellation.

'Vagina man' is a type of male hysteric who seeks affiliation with the maternal order in opposition to the paternal order. As such, he fulfils the wish of all hysterics, to decline the arrival of the father and to seek a renegotiated and more intense bond with the mother, either by adoration or by identification.

If the hysteric mother declines the primal scene by, as mentioned, refusing to include the father in all sorts of ways, we may see how the hysteric father achieves the same in his dismantlings of his function. Indeed, in the above clinical extract, the father actually projected his function into his wife, to whom he and the children looked for paternal structure, which she obligingly supplied.

The father's refusal to take up his symbolic function is a highly complex family reality, one that will bear on our subsequent discussion of the differences between the borderline, the hysteric and the perverse characters. It is perhaps best to keep in mind that such fathers, when they are 'good enough', instantiate into their bearing another form of 'anti-hysteria', inoculating their children against the otherwise malign effect of their positions. They often convey to their children not only a sense, but even a clear outline, of the 'failed father' or the 'loopy father', which in the dialectical imagination brings to the child's mind the imagined opposite. They may, indeed, prove to be gentle and fragile creatures who convey to their children a true sense of regret that they have failed to come together into the grown-up self.

The child of such a father puts it well.

> My father was one of the most generous people I have ever known. He would take everyone out to dinner and loved to tell stories and get others to do the same. He knew hundreds of jokes and was verbally very affectionate, always telling one person or the next how gifted or clever they were. Even if it was a bit of an act – because at home he could be quite a sort of collapsed guy, hardly the bonhomie of his outings – it was still part of what we took to be him, and we loved him for it. But he was so childlike. Not in a simpering way, but almost totally in a body way. For example, in adolescence I noticed for the first time that whenever he was introduced to a man whom he did not know he either hid or he performed a kind of little jig, like a kid meeting a cricket hero. His voice elevated, he giggled a lot, and he perspired profusely. Or at home, whenever we had to face a family issue – simple things like planning a holiday or more complicated like facing certain economic problems – he would joke and joke and try to get us to laugh our way out of it, or, he would momentarily assume differing types of adult characters – sometimes putting different voices to them – which annoyed the hell out of us, but which was also a little scary, as he would insist that he was who he was and that we were rotters for getting at him. He was sweet, but chaotic.

To sum up, then, both the mother and the father may decline their functions and, as hysterics, do so through subtle forms of absenteeism from their own sexuality and their responsibility for bearing and transmitting it. Confusing as this might be for the children, some hysterical parents mock themselves and invite the children to build sexual models elsewhere. One hysterical parent may project his or her function into the other non-hysterical parent, for example, when a mother might pass on the function of body erotisation to the father, or when the father might pass off the function of his law-making to the mother. If both parents are hysterics, then as a couple they may invite their children's mockery in order to help the children move on in life and not make the same errors as they did. If so, there is a genuinely self-sacrificial quality to such mockery, which, even though it serves other functions, is also of true help to the children who seek parental guidance. Later we will consider parents and children who create hysterical families, and in the next chapter we turn to the issue of seduction and abuse.

It remains to be emphasised, however, that the mother and the father are always the foremost psychic structures to any self. Akin to the self's determination of inner processes that will be derived (in part) from the actual mother's or actual father's way of being and relating, inner structures also derive from a culture's transmission of its own interpretation of maternal and paternal orders, as well as the child's idiomatically shifting mental tendencies over the early months and years of life. In limiting ourselves to the hysteric, we find someone whose internal father is a weakened structure, a compromise between differing glimpses of him as useless either by virtue of idealisation or by virtue of denigration, but which will be engaged on the level of the false self and, to varying or lesser extents, exploited to some gain. Just as the hysteric was never sure of the mother's desire for the self's sexuality, the hysteric is never sure of the father's solidity as a figure who would separate the child from the mother under cover of the promise of maturational accomplishment.

This instability owes as much to the hysteric's determination to undermine the function of the father as it does to any intrinsic weakness in the father, but we cannot conclude this chapter – and this part of the book – without an important caveat.

If the hysteric has suffered maternal cancellation of the self's sexual promise, then however much this would predispose the self toward hysteria, the father can mitigate this tendency by right of his symbolic function as the family inseminator; that is to say, in his function as upholder of the phallus (here interpreted as a function that bars the self from the mother in order to empower the self in its progression) the father symbolises his desire for the child's sexual progression. Even if the child is partly seeking to eradicate the implications of his or her own sexuality, if the father adequately conveys his desire for the child's eventual realisation of the child's sexuality, then he can assist the child in the erotisation of the future, rather than leave the child to the hysteric's inevitable erotisation of the past. No more should be said about this, however, to avoid the danger of creating a kind of schematic organisation for the hysteric, suggesting a single, fixed or predetermined pathway for all the character disorders envisioned by psychoanalysis. Fortunately, there are just too many variables in any individual's psychic reality for this to be the case. The self's psychic history involves everything we have discussed and any one self's solution will have been arrived at in a unique ordering, even if the self shares with many others – as we all do – well-known classes of psychic conflict.

Note

1   See Adam Phillips's brilliant essay 'Looking at Obstacles', in *On Kissing Tickling and Being Bored* (1993).

Chapter 7

The seduction of the story

As described in Chapter 4, the ordinary mother finds breast-feeding to be an intense erotic communication with her infant. If she is at ease with a new-found pleasure (that is yet archaic and instinctually based) she will communicate to the infant her pleasure in the infant as an erotic being. There is a type of lust in the breast to be suckled that meets with an increasing lust in the infant to suck, and this initial intercourse is deeply fulfilling to both figures, who achieve a type of mutual orgasm, the infant going off to sleep, the mother glowing in the after-bliss.

Freud pointed out that the infant discovers the independent nature of sexuality-in-itself in the pleasure of thumb-sucking: he or she does not need the breast to enjoy the pleasure of sucking. This leads to the foundation of infantile auto-erotism, but interestingly, the mother often intervenes by exchanging auto-erotic objects. She sucks her baby's fingers, just as she offers her own finger for sucking, thus consecrating the auto-erotic object with maternal libido. The infant who sucks his or her thumb alone sucks an object the mother has sucked, linking auto-erotism with allo-erotism.

The mother's seductions are a most subtle art. She coos about the infant's 'poo', seducing her baby into giving up wanton anal evacuation pleasures for the sensation of anal control linked to the fulfilment of maternal desire. 'Now that's a gooooooood girl', or 'Whaaaat a gooooood boy', chortles mum when the child lets her know that he or she wants to do a poo, finding that retention in this instance produces a *Liebestod* from the mother.

Originally Freud thought that a child sexually molested before puberty would not have sufficient mental grasp of the event to comprehend it and would only experience a fright but not a thinking of the fright. After puberty, when the child's genital mental representations had been comprehended more fully, he or she might then feel the mental effect of what had happened, if he or she had been subject to molestation at an earlier age. This recollection would de-repress the original trauma accompanied by the affect.

Freud discovered that all prior events – including non-sexual happenings – could become sexualised, a part of his theory of *Nachträglichkeit*, which Strachey translated as 'deferred action', whilst the French speak of '*après coup*', and Laplanche of 'afterwardness'. As this concept broadened, it included the effect of any prior psychic event in present lived reality that served to evoke it. But if we think of the effects of adolescent sexuality on the child self, all children will – to a lesser or greater extent – also retrospectively[1] sexualise the past. Adolescence might, of course, be the occasion for a massive de-repression of a former sexual molestation, one which means that the self is likely to be overwhelmed either by the memory, or in a kind of intrapsychic echo, by the charge of that trauma upon the present moment.

A child may sexualise the non-sexual. For example, an adolescent boy of 16 has several memories of his childhood that have been pleasant ones: at 4, sitting on his father's lap watching a football match; at 6, sitting with his mother in a jacuzzi for a few minutes of bliss; at 8, fishing in a boat with his uncle. At 16, however, now that he is much more aware of bodies and their sexualities, it briefly occurs to him that of course the father's lap was an area of the father's genitals. He recalls his mother in a bathing costume, and now sees the shape of her body rather differently. He has read about children being molested by uncles, cousins and other relatives, and the thought crosses his mind that maybe this was why the uncle took him fishing that day. These ideas and other retrospective investments will usually be unconscious or preconscious and will not go anywhere; that is, they will not strike the self as believable. Not, that is, unless the child is part of an epidemic of suspicion, such as exists especially in certain areas of England and North America, where a child undergoing an ordinary retrospection might suddenly believe that it happened. Perhaps he would tell a brother or a sister and in a short period of time, these projections of sexuality into non-sexual past events would then be passed on from one person to the next.

Let us return to the theory of *Nachträglichkeit* and to the particular period of time that is an object of emphasis in our study of the hysteric: the child's experience of the mother and the father around about the age of 3. Sexuality is disruptive and projectively identified into the father, whose job it is to bear this act of riddance.

At the same time, this father may be the first real thinking of the mother who was sexually disruptive and who is experienced as intrusive. During this period and the oedipal stage to follow, the child's complex attitude toward the father includes the first remembering of the early mother. Paternal disruptiveness, his disapproval of certain naughty behaviours, elicits memories of the disapproving mother. Indeed, all those traumata – in the sense of ordinary shocks to the self's experience of its own sanguine grandiosity – that were experienced before knowledge of the unwanted, intrusive other was discovered are now able to be thought through the name of the father.

Ironically, then, the father's arrival serves a curiously welcome function. Thinking about him and his intrusions allows the child to think out maternal intrusiveness. Thinking about sexuality through him allows the child to remember maternal sexuality.

Now the child thinks through the mother-as-other for the first time. Indeed, 'the third', which is held in the name of the father, allows the child to remember the mother as third object. But how could the exemplar of the dyadic other be at the same time a third object?

As a figure who desires in her own right, whose desire, although partly encompassing her infant, is independent of the infant's needs, as the figure who has her own internal conflicts, her own private set of ambitions exclusive of her interest in her child, *this* mother always existed somewhere outside the domain of the holding environment. This mother-on-the-outside existed beyond the dyad and indicated her status as a third object. She may be the bearer of the maternal order, but she has long since been an active participant in the fulfilment of those desires realising themselves through the paternal order.

The father inherits and sustains the mother's status as a prior third object, and if the child can negotiate this father, he or she also simultaneously encounters and processes the maternal third: maternal aggression, maternal desire, maternal self-interests. In part, the oedipal father is maternal afterwardness, when what was experienced but incapable of representation is now thought for the first time, through the figure and the function of the father.[2]

In 'Three Essays' (1905b) Freud writes of the nursing mother that she 'herself regards him with feelings that are derived from her sexual life' and that she 'treats him as a substitute for a complete sexual object' (p. 223). In a series of compelling and challenging essays, Jean Laplanche (1992) argues that maternal sexuality is communicated to the infant and, because her unconscious is formed and the child's is not, she becomes a compelling enigma that forces the infant to try to answer the question 'What does the breast want of me?' This is so, I believe, for all infants, just as the hysteric's later question 'Who am I as object in mother's internal world?' is also true of all people.

What cures the infant of maternal erotisation of his or her body and the breast-feed? It is the infant's own instinct (not *Trieb*), driven from his or her own primal fantasy. The erotic object (breast) is the joint erotic object of two thoughtless lovers.

For the normal infant this erotic bond is the foundation of the self's being, and the deferred action of infantile intercourse with the mother will express itself throughout life fundamentally in erotic moments. Its first traumatic after-effect is when the 3-year-old child, due to biological surge, now realises maternal erotism. Of course, it has been present all along, but only now – afterwards – is it gaining its first thinking. As Laplanche stresses, the mother becomes an 'enigmatic signifier' and this after-effect is traumatic. For the hysteric it is the occasion when the self feels divorced from the sexual, as if the child hears echoed from the past 'I told you so', linking the child's alienation from his or her body with the mother's prior alienation from his or her sexual body. It is only now, in this marriage between two separate eras of sexual renunciation, that hysteria as a point of character fixation is in a position to be created.

The non-hysteric, too, feels the shock of the self's sexuality and the mother's erotism being thought now for the first time. But this child also has the dynamic trace of his or her own instinct, just now also having its own *Nachträglichkeit*, so that from the history of his or her instinct comes renewed lust for mamma as sex object, an after-effect that propels the child on to the oedipal stage.

Unsurprisingly, many mothers are shocked by the erotic nature of breast-feeding. Matters are not helped by the fact that nursing mothers constitute a ghetto culture, profoundly neglected by Western societies. Even women who enjoy breast-feeding find it difficult to say so to other nursing mothers; rarely do books on mothering address this pleasure, and it is uncommon for doctors or postnatal caretakers to discuss it either. And all mothers have powerful psychic reasons to forget this moment in their lives – a few years later they will have only dim memories of this particular erotic relationship.

Many mothers are in fact horrified by their erotic response to suckling and abandon it abruptly. One need not enumerate the many negative responses; it is sufficient to make the point that such maternal revulsion will be communicated to the infant right at the beginning – and when the child of 3 finds his or her sexuality disruptive, erotism once again ruptures the relation to the mother, evoking unconscious memories of maternal rejection of their mutual erotism. Projecting the structure of this rupture into the father helps the child to unconsciously objectify the original trauma, although now it will be restaged with the father as the necessary embodiment of the horrors of sexuality.

With the acceptance of the sexual mother, however, comes a corresponding acceptance of the self's own sexuality, now conferred upon the self's prior sexual states. What is rather crudely thought of as 'pre-oedipal' sexuality – the instinctual realisations through erogenous zones and their sprung mental objects – is only fully thinkable in the oedipal period; indeed, this is the first thinking of prior existence and the psycho-sexual conflicts of the early years of life are never more finely represented than they are through the structure of the oedipal triangle.

Oedipus thinks his early days through his encounter with the complex that confronts him in Thebes. The lesson of Sophocles, as with the theory of *Nachträglichkeit*, is that the past is available for its proper thinkings in the later course of human life, so much so that we may wonder if the term *Nachträglichkeit* should not stand for the very character of human development. Are we not always just translating something known but not thought, through the course of life events and psychic changes that permit us to think our knowledge for the first time?

As we shall see, however, the hysteric does not use the oedipal period for sexual translation. At best, he or she seeks to be in limbo between two countervailing options: as a transcendent asexual self or as a precocious sexual false self. To some extent, the hysteric does and does not accept the father, does and does not retrospectively sexualise the mother, and does and does not inherit the self's desire. The hysteric will oscillate in life between hot and cold, passion and indifference, as he or she moves into and out of sexual desire.

As Gregorio Kohon writes, hysterics do not know their own gender. Being in limbo means being both a boy and a girl – but, we might add, a boy and a girl of immature genitalia, refusing further mental elaboration of genitals, without a retrospective sexualisation of the mother and of the self, and therefore without a true acceptance of the function of the father.

In the more extreme forms of hysteric character formation, driven by the death instinct, there is a different type of *Nachträglichkeit*: the after-effects of maternal decathexis (part of the work of repression), which the infant experiences as a petrification of the self. Oftentimes, idealisation is the mortar of such petrifaction, seeking to install rigidly secure objects in the place of libido. Not uncommonly, this hysteric will seek a type of monastic isolation or take a frozen anti-libidinal stance in the presence of others, a kind of violently desexualised virginity seeking to unsexualise the universe, by translating it into a transcendental sterilised community.

In this schizoid hysteria the self becomes stiff or stiffened, but unlike the schizoid proper, the hysteric's aim is to freeze the sexual and to incarcerate desire in a monastic stance. The schizoid, experiencing the mother as deeply offended by the child's bodily being, imagines and comes to regard his or her body as a kind of faecal mass. Believing that he or she was excreted from the mother's behind, the schizoid feels she is loath to touch the child with love and, owing to his or her own aversion to the mother's body and being, develops a contempt for the body and its needs. The hysteric's conflict with the body is not an anal one; the body is taken to be sexually offensive, not off-putting as an entire object in its own right. It is the body of intercourse and birth through the vaginal canal that brings up hysterical repulsion, whilst the schizoid offence is a kind of olfactory refusal of the body as stinker.

(The death-drive hysteric's specific hate of the sexual body may reflect a lifelong attack on intercourse: first, the mother's erotic intercourse with the self, then parental intercourse, then the self's relation to the other. Envy of maternal erotism drives the turn to auto-erotic solutions which paralyse the mother. Still this mother presents herself as exciting and the child cannot yet go into the monastery and must eliminate his or her erotism through self-stimulation, serving the death instinct. In milder form, this is the adult who masturbates not out of desire, but proactively to get rid of emergent excitement.)

To some extent the hysteric suffers an auto-trauma. The refusing oedipal child who retrospectively petrifies the self and its others freezes the libidinal self inside a particular character stance that becomes a self-inflicted trauma. Religious hysterics who flagellate their bodies savagely deny their sexuality and only act out an existing petrifaction of the self's sexuality.

Nachträglichkeit has its own afterwardness. A second action may take place. In the wake of afterwardness may come retrospection: a present self's alteration of a past self's state, edited according to the terms of the present. For when we revise former selves we do not erase the prior version, we simply create a new edition, which lives alongside the prior self, rather like the way a painter might paint a series of paintings which, though similar, are new versions of the same image. Each time we subject a former self state to retrospection we create two selves: version one, version two.

This ordinary intrapsychic activity sponsors a temporal illusion that something has entered the space of the child and tampered with innocence. This someone is the later child, who challenges the status of the original version years later. As a paradigm operating throughout a person's life, an innocent version is always being threatened by a disturbing new one. Yet when the new vision is assimilated and taken as the truth, it then assumes its own totality, innocent of any other possible vision, until the next rendition, when the work of psychic life intrudes once again.

Nachträglichkeit is the nature of thought itself, especially if we separate afterwardness from retrospection. As our past psychic realities affect us, giving meaning to prior shocks only now coming fully to mind, not only is the past entering itself in the present, but the present self returns to its past inevitably creating new editions. As we are talking about psychic reality, afterwardness and retrospection often work alongside one another, even though they are very different mental phenomena.

Considering hysteria, we can see there is a double action that confers desire and anti-desire at the same time. Sexualisation is accompanied by petrifaction.

When the present self returns to a past self, the past self feels affected by something intruding from what it comprehends as its future. In considering the hysteric's sense of seduction and abuse we need to pay particular attention to the hysteric's experience of afterwardness–retrospection. It is as if the innocent self had been first libidinalised and then petrified. Or, to look at it descriptively, the person feels as if the visitation of sexuality is followed by the after-trauma of petrifaction.

A patient.

> All through my life I have had this underlying sense of being very innocent and pure. As a child – I think it was when I was nine or ten that I recall it – I would look at parts of my body, I remember especially my legs, and I would sort of smile at them and think that they were nice legs. I would wonder what it would be like, however, to grow up, to be a teenager and then an adult. I knew I would change, but I thought to myself that my body would still be itself, that my leg, with its particular moles and other features would be a constant. I also thought a lot about who I was at the time. I promised myself that I would remember how important I was to myself in that moment, that I would never forget, and that I would never look back with anything like contempt or disapproval on my self at that moment. I would look about the room at a newspaper or something with a date on it and I would promise myself that I would always remember that date and that moment. But I think when only a few months passed all these moments would be forgotten.
>
> But I also remember feeling that so called 'developmental firsts' like the first time I had facial hair, the first time I had a specific sexual erection, the first time I made out with a girl, the first time . . . you know all these firsts . . . I felt a strange sense of loss and of violation. I thought I lost my innocence and my

purity and in some way I felt each of these 'milestones' was a violation of myself. I don't want to exaggerate, because at the same time, another part of me was pleased, but it was not a situation without some real conflict.

No sooner, however, would I settle into a next phase of my life – whether I was in a new town, in a new job, with a new lover, or whatever – when my immediate self would seem innocent again and any change would strike me as violating that innocence. It got to the point when just before coming to see you, when I would go into a bookstore to just browse and find a new work by a new author, instead, when I passed by authors whose works I loved and had become part of my innocent self, I would feel I had to buy one of their works – which I usually did – and I would then re-read a book which I had read many times over. For example, I think I have fifteen different versions of *The Mill on the Floss* which I have read almost every year of my life since I was a teenager.

This man sought analysis in his thirties, and his description partly illuminates that hysterical loyalty to one's innocent self. To an extent, what he describes is common to all of us. He was not severely disturbed, but he was aware of a boyish resistance to new experiences in life which he could not understand. His wife complained about his 'boring sexual techniques' as he only made love in the missionary position, which he saw as 'innocent'. Anything more adventurous struck him as 'deviant', even 'dirty'.

As *Nachträglichkeit* is an instrumental feature in the psychic development of the self, the hysteric is often averse to life encounters which evoke revisions. There is a fear of unconscious participation in life. New experiences release old – latent – desires and conflicts which, if activated, would push the hysteric out of the simple boy or girl self and compel them towards adult life.

As a compromise the hysteric seeks correlates to life experience which allow for vicarious proceedings that in some respects are powerful but are contained and well defended against. An example would be literary experience, when used to fill in for life, so that the sexual and emotional adventures in the novel effect a specular self: as the reader, a step removed. In this way, the equivalent of any past self may be brought into the present in the form of the reader's mentality. The hysteric controls the experience of reading, dosing the self as he or she can refuse to turn the page, or can put the novel down until a more suitable moment. Psychic realisations are safer because they are the creations of the text and the self is not so personally affected.

A patient in her late thirties had been very withdrawn during her twenties, only going out of her house to work, and returning to a flat that was monastic. She never socialised and took refuge in countless novels, videos and tending to her cats. She read a novel about a woman who was not unlike herself, and the character in the story took a cookery course which enabled her to invite guests to sumptuous meals. So she did the same. Indeed, she became a remarkable gourmet and invited friends from work to Saturday evening meals. She bought a long pine table to seat twelve people, very elegant place settings and cutlery, and she procured fine wines. As these events were extraordinary hits she expanded her list and looked forward to her dinners with true pleasure. Her dinner guests assumed, she reckoned, that she had a very active life, yet they would have been surprised to find that during the week she was a recluse. When she held her parties she felt that she stepped into someone else's skin.

The finding of the hysterical intermediate self, between the true self and the social order, is an important part of the hysteric's search for a place. He or she seeks to create a self capable of this sort of life experience and from here may actually venture out into the world practising a kind of applied literature.

The evolution of this false self may be deeply unconscious and the application of a fantasy self upon lived experience may be more subtle than in the above case. A man in his late twenties, for example, had lived his life celebrating what he regarded as his eccentricity. He had a fairly common name – something like Frederick Compton – and he called himself 'FC', as did his friends. He wore bow ties and braces from late adolescence and refused certain foods, such as chicken, broccoli, salmon and hamburgers, whilst relishing others, such as lamb chops, spinach, veal and hot dogs. All who knew him the least bit well discovered his culinary likes and dislikes and this was something that one had to accommodate around FC. He drove his car giving hand signals rather than using the indicator; he bought vinyl records during the CD era; and he became an expert on peonies, which he grew in his garden. He had a distinctive walk; when he talked he often raised his right eyebrow, and he would take his hat off every few minutes, wipe the inside rim with his handkerchief, and put it back on. To these traits one could add hundreds of other notable characteristics and certainly many of his friends thought that FC was 'something else'.

Unfortunately, FC had unconsciously constructed these oddities in order to delight a split-off observing part of him that would say, 'Isn't he cute?' Being cute was, he realised, an important part of being FC and his last girlfriend would punctuate their conversations every few minutes with an 'Oh, FC, you are outrageous', which delighted him.

FC knew, however, that his eccentricities were not spontaneous, not from the true self – but adoptions from books, movies and premeditated character inventions that appealed to him. There were very few links between his eccentric manners and his inner life. As he discovered in analysis, he was an invention of a part of himself that wished to admire a cute little boy and get others to enter into the circle of admiration.

To an extent FC was seduced by the pleasures of being the cute little boy who always gained the surprise and rapture of adults. He was a pure delight to his mother, who worshipped him. He amused her endlessly with 'actings' – when he would portray a family friend or a TV character, or a certain stereotypical figure like a southern American or a New Yorker – and when he came across a character in a book he read or a film he watched or even when he met someone who impressed him, he would later on 'act them out'. As discussed in Chapter 3, hysterics derive an ability to get into stories which they then enact because they have been driven to find themselves in the mother's internal world. As they develop the mother's negatives they become skilled in this particular act of development.

They are drawn to enact the unconscious preoccupations of a society. As the literature of abuse is one of our most compelling stories, the scene of seduction becomes a type of imaginary place that uncannily captures aspects of the hysteric's original psychic paralysis. Except now the hysteric is being seduced by stories – stories of seduction. The agent of trauma is not the happening itself but the other's account of the happening.

We may recall the mother who shies away from touching her infant's body and who substitutes voice and narrative for physical stimulation and mutually developed inter-erogeneity. Being seduced by the story recalls a type of maternal seduction in which the story of the self and other fills in for the engaged erotics of self and other.

A patient.

> I did not like going to school very much. But I loved hearing from one of my friends about what happened at school that day. It was always better to hear about it than to actually experience it. If only I could have had this friend tell me a story about school and maybe a teacher send me books and exams, I think I could have done well there, but the place itself was pretty dreadful.

Some hysterics become intensely interested in telling their story. But the telling is their living, so the repeated telling of the story is needed in order to keep the self and its others alive where they live: in the story. Often superb narrators, they may enter the story of abuse and tell it with greater skill and charm than those who have actually suffered from sexual abuse. This should not be surprising. In Hollywood an entire industry of experts has developed the capacity to get inside the other's character. Any skilled actor can portray an ordinary person's life far better than the ordinary person could. Much of the literature of abuse, whether written by a therapist or a recovering victim or both, reads like adolescent romantic fiction.

As a gifted *identifier* and *representer* the hysteric often tells the story of the self and its others with remarkable dramatic impact. Like the mother who unconsciously seduces the child into the story of the child – either an inner story 'told' silently to an internal object or an actual serial telling of the mother's desire – the hysteric seduces his or her others into a captive belief that in some respects violently repudiates the notion of the illusory. The hysteric may present a theme to the analyst – sexual fear, despair, suicide – but it is not meant to be examined; it is intended to capture the analyst through the power of the image. It is not meant to be thought about, because the action of scrutiny and interpretation introduces its own brand of afterwardness and the hysteric demands to be taken at face value. If unconscious themes are explored the hysteric will act out (and in) in an effort to force the analyst to return to the manifest presentation (the innocent or pure scene), not sullying this truth with reconsideration.

Insistence on the manifest presentation may be violent. The hysteric who threatens suicide sometimes does so to prove to the analyst that the story should never have been questioned in the first place. If the spectral self operating inside its applied literature is threatened, he or she may take revenge by saying, through suicide, 'I will show you how this is my truth and prove to you that you should never have sought anything other than the manifest text.' In the imaginary, the hysteric lives on after death, witnessing his or her funeral. The hysteric does not want to die – in the midst of this theatre he or she does not comprehend that a staged suicide ends in death. For the hysteric it is simply one of life's most powerful stories and the lure to act it is a constant temptation.

Eventually, the analyst confronts the hysteric's near addiction to living as a character within his or her own story. All along, the hysteric has unconsciously erotised narrative. The self was always an erotic object inside the other's discourse, and this is adopted by the hysteric, who, developing an auto-erotic reverie as compensation for the comparative absence of maternal sensorialisation, over-invests the self and its objects in the world of fantasy. By adult life the hysteric's narrations are themselves auto-erotic reveries, whilst internal processes of thought are medleys of excitations, romantic imaginings, yearnings and pinings, and grudges against the real world.

In psychoanalytic sessions the hysteric's free associations not uncommonly begin to serve a sexual function, as the patient's wordings conjure topics of excitement which conclude in hysterical orgasm. A patient, sensing that he or she is wandering into an interesting area of discourse, is stimulated by his or her own speech and 'comes' in language when his or her interest has been exhausted. The comparative flatness of subsequent associations are post-orgasmic wordings, expressing the self's decathexis of language as erotic stimulation. Typically, the patient then forages through topics, often memories of the previous day's events, in the hope that one topic will carry a latent sexual excitation which would then be exploited to serve up another speech-orgasm. It will be recalled that the hysteric's sexual body has been displaced to language itself, and it is through speaking – especially passionately so – that the hysteric feels his or her erotic life has been articulated and met by the other. It really is, in some ways, through the ear.

Analytic interpretation of the hysteric's narrations is ipso facto unwelcome. As an appreciative listener and witness, all is fine. As one who would intervene in the story, to suggest other possible scenes and understandings, the analyst imperils auto-erotic reverie with the implicit demands of an 'intercourse' between two intimates. Of course, this conflict is analysable, and finally there is no alternative to simply speaking this to the hysteric, but amongst the resistances facing the analyst is the hysteric's true sense of uncertainty about the outcome of such an invitation. If he or she feels the narrative self will not be accepted, admired, loved and adored as is, but instead challenged in any way, then the hysteric may commit suicide to preserve the purity of his or her eros. On the other hand, the intrusion of inter-pretation may elicit an erotic craving for the analyst, a desperate effort to assimilate the otherness of the analyst through auto-erotic management. The insistence that the analyst will eventually prove a true love object is all the time an illusion, as it sustains a form of loving and pining that was never intended to move out of its auto-erotic base.

More commonly, it is at the point of analytical engagement of the patient's relation to his or her own narrated self that the hysteric often suggests a reduction in sessions or an end to treatment. By seeking a reduction in sessions the patient tries to coerce the analyst into 'backing off' and, if the analyst agrees and actually reduces the number of hours, the possibility of 'breaking' the patient's auto-erotic circuit is diminished.

(The death-drive hysteric seeks total silence, his or her narrations of life kept secret, unspoken. To talk is to engage in a form of intercourse. The other is not to receive this pleasure. Instead, the other is to yearn for contact, and on occasion believe it is occurring, only to find it dashed. To talk to the analyst is to betray the death work[3] which is opposed to representation, except for the continued picturing of the self as doing without the realisation of the body's desire.)

The strength of the hysteric's auto-erotism cannot be overstated. As it was Fairbairn who concentrated on this particular aspect of hysteria, we now turn to his theories and to further consideration of auto-erotic reveries.

Notes

1 As John Fletcher (1999) points out in his excellent introduction to Jean Laplanche's book *Essays on Otherness*, *Nachträglichkeit* and retrospection are not one and the same process. Afterwardness refers to the effect of a sexual event in later life as it occurs in the changing temporal contexts. Retrospection refers to the reconstruction of past events according to the sexuality of the present. Even though these terms are different, I shall include both ideas in the area surrounding the word *Nachträglichkeit* because an important part of my theory is based on the understanding that the self will experience the after-effects of its infantile sexuality throughout life.

2 This may help explain why psychoanalysis – depending on the theorist – differs over who threatens the child with castration and who possesses the phallus: mother or father. We would have to say both, but ultimately anxiety over castration and the fear of the holder of the phallus will be associated with the father's name, as it is through engagement with the oedipal father that the child fully conceptualises his or her anxieties.

3 'Death work' is a term coined by J.-B. Pontalis (1981) in his essay 'On death work'.

Chapter 8

Hot and cold

According to Fairbairn (1954), the first defence used by 'the original ego' is the alliance with 'an unsatisfying personal relationship', which constitutes an introjection of the 'unsatisfying object' (p. 15). This unsatisfactory state consists of an object that 'has two disturbing aspects, viz. an exciting aspect and a rejecting aspect' (p. 16). The hysteric's object is both excessively exciting and excessively rejecting.

Fairbairn believes that the exciting and the rejecting aspects of the object are split off by the ego, forming three objects: (1) the exciting, (2) the rejecting and (3) the nucleus that remains (relatively satisfying).

The rejection and splitting off constitute a primary and secondary repression. In addition, a central ego remains to cathect an ideal object that is acceptable, whilst the two other objects are repressed and cathected by portions of the ego that structure them. The 'libidinal ego' goes with the exciting object and the 'antilibidinal ego' goes with the rejecting object.

Fairbairn's hysteric poses a conflict in his relations that derives from an object. The hysteric who is overly exciting presents such a self to the other, only later to present an overly rejecting self. Or an overly rejecting self may flip into an overly exciting self: a classic example of the teasing–rejecting side of the hysteric. Following Fairbairn, however, we must assume that this pairing affects each of its individual splits, so the exciting self suggests its opposite, as does the rejecting self. Indeed, we know that in the love scene a rejecting self may point to its denied excitement, leading the other to sense that what is wanted is transportation to the zone of excitement. This would be momentary fusion by force of the other. It is sadly ironic that such a search is unconsciously apt, as it was the self's experience that the maternal environment seemed to occasion this split. Now the hysteric seeks an other to forcefully end the split, restoring a unified ego.

Although the hysteric does not intend his or her sexuality to be realised, his or her offer and then rejection, may be mistaken as sincere, especially when it operates in the sexual field. Furthermore, although the hysteric may be having sexual intercourse regularly, he or she does so from a frame of mind subtly dissociated from the sexual act, operated by the central ego that functions in a magically manipulative manner. That is, the central ego knows that it can move from one extreme to the other and yet if these two poles cancel one another out, then a relatively sane self is left. When moving into the love space the hysteric does so as a magic realist, the elements of excitement and rejection often juggled before the eyes of the other. The manipulator self survives by cultivating its magical power in order to diminish the work of the other sectors of the self.

A homosexual patient.

> I would drive my lovers crazy, I mean really drive them mad. Because when I would pick them up I would be in a spell of the erotic, really into being sexual, and . . . I was bait, boy was I bait. I got carried away by it, off on it. And a lover would take me off with him, but when we got to the place to fuck, something else overcame me . . . a sort of, well, an odd feeling that I was also on the verge of sainthood. Don't ask me why, because I have no idea. But it was as if my lover's desire for me changed me, or I felt this change into something pure. And when he undressed me, which I always insisted upon, I would go back and forth in my own mind – and with my lover – between states of sexy frenzy and the absolute opposite: states of sainthood. If you could have seen the look on their faces.

For Fairbairn (1954) the central ego may have an ideal object that is sexless. This excludes the sexual and the rejecting, but with the analyst in the transference although there is an effort to control the situation through exclusion, the erotic transference will break this down. Fairbairn describes two patients, Louise and Morris, whose hysteria is the outcome of parents who were exciting and rejecting. Later, when discussing hysteria as madness, we will return to the potential effect of such parenting, but Fairbairn's virtually exclusive focus on the parent's actual behaviour is too extreme and, ironically, refuses the conflict with the sexual.

For with the recognition of sexuality at 3, the child (not the parents) refuses these two elements – excitability and rejection – by projecting them into the mother and the father. This leaves a sexless self aiming to form a relation to an ideal object that is itself sexless; this, as we know, is the effort of the hysteric to transcend (manically, precociously, by identification not assimilation) genitality.

However, Fairbairn's focus on the role of the parent is an important one. As discussed in previous chapters, each hysteric experiences failed maternal libidinalisation of his or her body. If the mother is excited by her baby, she cannot directly translate it into bodily confirming touch. There is a re-routing of maternal desire through several stages. First, she dissociates herself from physical confirmation of her infant's genitals, then she constitutes an erotic baby within her internal world and proceeds in her auto-erotic reveries to make love to that internal body. In touching the actual baby's body, she can convey something of that erotism, but it will be displaced from the genitals – which are always objects of maternal avoidance – to other parts of the body, now treated as erotic objects. The body, however, is touched as if it were a corporeal materialisation of her own internal object, overdetermined further by the fact that in touching it she carries both the aversive energy of dissociation and the intense embrace of a highly cathected libidinal object. The infant will come to understand himself or herself as the carnal realisation of the mother's erotic life, stifled when it reaches the genitalia, but polymorphously active and the object of intense narrative and performative interest, guided by maternal auto-erotism.

When sexuality becomes a trauma at 3, separating the self from the mother, it may recall an earlier conflict when the mother experienced the infant's sexuality as divisive. The infant bears this maternal interpretation of sexuality, which becomes a predisposition to the later shock at 3 when sexuality is once again disruptive.

In cancelling out the sexual, the child joins maternal cancellation and marries the non-sexual or anti-sexual aspects of the mother, who creates erotic objects only in the internal world. The child feels authorised from the maternal order. Indeed, the child feels an uncanny marriage with the mother's rejection of the sexual at the point when sexuality seems to disrupt the child's world. An unconscious contract of sorts is signed, in which it is agreed that sexuality and the body debase the purer aims and lives of the self. A sacrifice takes place, as the rejection of the body is one's own bodily being and one's own sexual attractiveness. The reward is the marriage of mother and child, who sacrifice engaged erotism to a higher and purer love of one another, driven by auto-erotism.

In two further cases described by Fairbairn – Jean and Olivia – he argues that there was probably a 'prematurely stirred' (1954: 25) genitality and he wonders about the intrusions of the parent. As ambivalent action would have it, we may assume that the mother's ambivalence toward the genitalia – especially the negative side – unconsciously exposes an excitement, an erotisation, which is allowed to live on as the sexualisation of refusal, or what André Green means by 'the negative' (1998). When Fairbairn (1954) goes on to say that the hysteric uses auto-erotism as a compensation for the absence of closeness, he fails to see that through auto-erotics the child recognises desire of the mother, to achieve gratification onanistically and not with the other: to find through the internal object the erotic object of desire, evoked by touching the self. This erotic object is uncontaminated by the failures of the other, who will not fit into the grandiose script.

Furthermore, the other's actual touch breaks the auto-erotic circuit. It shocks the hysteric, who never intended the other to engage the self sexually (unless the other can quickly and secretly be adopted as if it were a part of the self, so the other's genital is used as a masturbatory tool in an auto-erotic act).

As the hysteric's internal objects are kept alive by auto-erotic libido, there is an erotic base to inner imagining: the everyday becomes charged with sexuality. The hysteric, however, maintains an affective indifference to the charge of the objects, often drawing the analyst into interpretation of the sexual innuendo but appearing quite removed.

Fairbairn would see this as a conflict between the libidinal and anti-libidinal self. To which we may add that when the narrative contents are excited, the narrative delivery is often cold; and when the narrative delivery is cold, the contents are libidinal. That is to say, the conflict is usually between the container and the contained, with one or the other being the libidinal or the anti-libidinal, another aspect of the hysteric's sexual anguish.

Think of it again in terms of the infant–mother relation. The mother handles (i.e. contains) the infant's genital libidinal body with anti-libido but erotically celebrates the non-genital body parts. In slightly dissociated fashion, the infant experiences this divisive and diversionary maternal desire with curiosity. He or she sees mother's libido in action but it is demonstrated *on* rather than *with* the infant.

This is a displacement created by the mother. The child grasps objects that are anti-libido with passion and offers the self as an anti-libidinal object, because as such it may be passionately embraced.

This is very often a matter of gaze. It is as if the self says 'I offer my self as an ornament of sexual attractiveness (anti-libido) and you may embrace the sight, but you cannot touch the object.' As the mother's desire is solely directed towards her internal objects, the hysteric tries to be loveable, performing those objects in her presence. The child wishes to be carried off as her introject, serving the pleasures of her memory, sustained by the self's own erotic devotion to the maternal imaginary.

A patient.

> I am aware of being loveable to people and of giving them something through just being amusing and entertaining. I think it's also fair to say that people know that this is as far as it goes, as I rarely get from this sort of amusement any serious courtships from people. Perhaps . . . well, perhaps they know that I take pleasure in bringing up a laugh or being amusing and I hear back from friends in common how well I have been appreciated. I know that I am important in my so-called circle of friends. I think this is almost more important to me than actually meeting up with someone and establishing a long term relation, because I don't know what to do with an actual lover. I think I am good story material for my friends. I hear back my tales, always changed a bit, on the grapevine. Its rather a lot of fun.

Fun it may be at times, but only by managing to push out of mind the very particular form of loss discussed in Chapter 6. By remaining childlike the hysteric banishes all those possible self states that otherwise would have evolved during the course of maturation. Although seeking compensation by deriving glowing smiles from admiring friends and living inside the other's storytelling worlds, the abandonment of true-self evolutions through the developing objects of life (school, sports, cultural quests, etc.) promotes a sense of the loss of true possibilities. The false self might indeed have gone on to excel in sports or school or cultural quests, but these 'successes' have always been grudgingly accomplished, against the wishes of the self. Even so, the hysteric grieves over the loss of the self that might have gone through life as a true rather than false expression of desire. Very often the hysteric breaks down in tears when touched, grieving the many losses of physical love. There is more to it, however.

There is a particular form of envy in the hysteric. Often preoccupied with what others have gone on to accomplish, the hysteric envies the other's maturational process, not simply what the other has accomplished. He or she fosters compensatory contempt towards the successful other often expressed in the view that such people have 'sold out' to the 'establishment'. Even when part of the establishment, the hysteric regards himself or herself as a true rebel and heaps private, if not public, scorn on those who take pleasure in their vocational and social progress.

This envy compounds hysterical loss. He or she continues to feed the truculent child who believes that going off with father sells out the pure self and its ideal other, inevitably the mother. The hysteric may disable himself or herself, either literally or figuratively, finding in disability a transcending nobility that renounces the ambitions of forward development.

One patient, quite successful in his career, felt he struggled for years to get ahead in life. Yet he always begrudged the parts of him that managed the success. Self envy[1] is common in the hysteric, who, ironically, envies the self's own capacities, since through acts of dissociation they are felt to be the property of the father: certainly not from the true self that aims to renew contact with the Madonna mother. The patient engaged in financially risky behaviour totally out of character with anything he had done before. In fact, he committed 'professional suicide', dismantling his professional status, losing his job, and throwing himself and his family into bankruptcy. The net effect of this castration was a period not only of great relief, but of manic celebration. He was, as he said, free at last, free at last.

For a time this seemed true. He took up fishing and sailing and pottery. He took a cookery course. His bewildered wife, faced with her husband's assertions that he was now in touch with his true self, tried to accept that the disasters they now confronted were essential. The four children – from latency through adolescence – were also perplexed, because although he was now giving them much more time than before, they were distressed by his apparent self abandonment and, of course, by the fact that there was no more money.

Fortunately, he entered analysis, where his complacent triumphalism was examined carefully and his self-damaging inclinations were analysed. His search to find some place of truth for himself was understood to be an important quest, but the oedipal dimensions of his conflict – risking the family's money to spit out his internal father and embrace a mother meant to love the pure boy in him – gave him a different perspective. He survived his 'suicide', rebuilt his business and home life, and fortunately found other means for achieving a lifestyle that suited him. And there were gains in all this. He became quite a good fisherman and his cookery skills brought some pleasure to the family.

The world is filled with less happy conclusions.

It is the hysteric who finds success a paradoxical accomplishment and aims to destroy it before matters go too far. It is the hysteric who defers socialisation by remaining childlike for as long as possible, sustaining the child self into his or her forties and fifties. If all the while he or she does indeed live with an acute sense that possibilities of the self have remained unfulfilled because of dalliance, the

hysteric may counter this by pointing to true accomplishments, and this charming
person is often gifted and productive. Still, this person knows that many creative
possibilities were squandered. He or she knows of personal relations that were
possible but neglected, in the interests of sustaining the boy or girl self who could
not be expected to sustain an adult's existence. The close friends of the hysteric are
more often than not left dumbfounded by how such a person can be so personally
(creatively and socially) wasteful: throwing away, neglecting or abandoning so
many forms of invigorated evolution. Such a sense of wastage is highlighted by the
hysteric's spurts of investment in life, which momentarily recuperate matters
to reveal a capability that only makes the subsequent spells of wastage even clearer.

As discussed in Chapter 3, the hysteric diverges from the path of normal
development charted by Freud, who regarded the castration complex as a pivotal
moment. As he saw it, the recognition by boys and girls of sexual difference, and
of the father's sexual 'ownership' of the mother and his law-making function,
prompted castration anxieties which led them to suspend desire for the mother. In
this symbolic castration, true desire must be repressed (a repression from which
paradoxically we all benefit), gratification must be postponed, and, because the
child must move from desire to identification, each gender increases its psychic
depth.

The hysteric, however, does not follow this course. He or she has experienced
sexuality itself as malignantly disruptive of the relation to the mother; and the
mother was never a proper sex object, but at best a passionately loved virginal
presence. For complex reasons, however, the hysteric develops a false self offered
to the father and his laws, apparently following a line of development that would
lead to postponement of sexual desire. It is crucial in understanding the hysteric,
however, to realise that he or she grows up in order to return to early pre-oedipal
desires. A clinical example will bring this into sharper focus.

By all accounts, Henry was a high-flyer who succeeded academically and
in athletics, eventually becoming a senior partner in a prestigious law firm. He
married and had two children, who were 10 and 8 respectively when he entered
analysis with a female clinician. In a startlingly brief period of time, Henry
regressed to a deeply idealising dependence and decided that he had had enough of
what he called the rat race and proposed to retire at 38. Over a course of months,
he told his analyst that ever since he was a child he could recall feeling that his
accomplishments were dictated more by a sense of anxiety than by any source of
pleasure. Henry recalled his father as an especially exacting man and he believed
that he excelled solely to keep his father 'off his back'. He had sexual affairs in his
early twenties and married a woman whom he thought he loved, but soon
afterwards lost his sexual appetite. He did, however, like his wife's company and
he loved both his children, although he felt increasingly that he was not 'up to
being a father'. In one session he told his analyst that he had only ever progressed
in life under the banner of a promise he had made to himself since late adolescence;
namely, that as soon as he had enough money, he would retire, and do what he
really wanted to do. When he entered analysis, the force of this promise surged to

the forefront of his mind, and for a long time he was determined to put this promise into practice.

This patient's form of hysteria is not at all unusual. Whilst the non-hysteric genuinely gets on with maturation, progressively enjoying work, love and play, the hysteric begrudges maturation itself. Unconsciously, it is perceived as the biologically imposed mandate that separated the self from the ideal world with the providing mother, and the self is determined to grow up in order to return to life as a child. These are people who almost always possess a 'bail-out' scene, a yearned-for moment promised to the self, when they can suddenly rid themselves of what are regarded as tediously intrusive responsibilities, and finally give themselves what they want. Paradoxically, the more successful they become as they enter mid-life, the more anxious they become, not because they fear castration by a father who will bar them from greater triumph, but because success further removes them from the mother to whom they are married.

In her theory of perversion, Janine Chasseguet-Smirgel maintains that the pervert seeks to return to the smooth world of the mother's belly, one devoid of any obstacles, especially those proposed by the paternal penis, or another sibling. The pervert regards obstacles of any kind as a hindrance to the longed-for return to untroubled existence, and to achieve this he or she subverts in differing ways the complex structures of life. There are similarities to the hysteric, but the hysteric's yearning to return to the mother is driven by complicated – fixed – identities that were commemorated in early childhood as forms of dedication to the desexualised

love object. Like the pervert, the hysteric seeks to substitute utopia for reality; but, unlike the pervert, the hysteric seeks to fulfil the other's desire, a drive which, ironically, compels the hysteric to sustain personal evolutions in relationships, culture and society, even as he or she yearns for the presumed opposite. It is as if the hysteric were saying to the mother, 'I promise to give myself to your desire', in the hope that he or she can then become the maternal love object; but after the oedipal stage, when this other now unwittingly includes the law of the father, the other replies, 'I accept your promise and my desire is that you give me your very best', a contract that drives the hysteric into his or her future, against the hysteric's own intrinsic wishes.

The hysteric's self-hate cannot be overestimated. The feeling that one has betrayed one's innocence by accepting participation in relations goes very deep and is one of the primary reasons why seriously depressed hysterics are always a high suicide risk.

One patient, who had been in hospital for some time and was quite ill when admitted, gradually got better in the course of her treatment. When she first arrived she was very deranged and childlike, but gradually she improved, and was well liked by other patients and the staff. There is no psychoanalyst who could, at the time, have seen how this would mandate a suicide, but looking back on this patient's suicide, the staff could see how her accomplishments were too precocious and her suicide was a killing-off of the hated part of her personality, which she felt had sold out her childhood.

It is the anorectic who most radically expresses the hysteric's ability to reverse the maturational process. Typically, this person is a precocious child who leap frogs into premature adulthood during adolescence, often attaining considerable academic success. It may not be until leaving school that he or she institutes the anorectic process. This anorectic's progressive loss of weight is only a corporeal manifestation of an evolving psychic reduction as the anorectic assumes a violent innocence in relation to his or her own self dismantling. The anorectic would have the other believe that he or she does not know the meaning of the weight reduction. Instead, he or she claims to have simply been caught up in the cultural bias toward the slim self, a childlike perspective that already constitutes a dismantling of this person's previously considerable intellect. The anorectic would have us believe that he or she is captive to a preoccupation with food and the body that was independent of a frame of mind – the return to being a child. Where psychodynamic was, the hysteric, as usual, invites an illness that is an overwhelming lure to the social unconscious. So universities have support groups for anorectics, which include 'support teams' composed of nutritionists, doctors and therapists who monitor blood pressure, diet and fear of food. Although these programs do save the lives of many anorectics, they do so, ironically, by colluding with the hysterical process, implicitly accepting the reduction of this complex adult into a simplified being. Where once the person was proud of his or her academic achievements, now he or she is proud of how much he or she eats and how good a patient he or she has become. Having opted out of the maturational path, the anorectic suggests a different progression, back to the good-boy or good-girl self (a crucial part of their childhood years) who pleases the support team, i.e. those adults who know how to treat this child. Alongside the anorectic are many others in this hysterical dismantling of the adult self, as others in the 'eating disorder' community, or those in the worlds of gamblers, drinkers, fornicators and 'workaholics' break down into new genres of disability with new teams of doctors and therapists springing up beside them like the towns that sprouted up along the newly constructed rail lines of the nineteenth century.[2]

One of the traits of the anorectic is the self's apparently hapless induction by a statement into a process that cannot be arrested. 'I said to myself that I could only eat one carrot at lunch and one piece of broccoli for dinner' – and so it shall be. By lowering the self's intellectual level to the place of one duped by language, the hysteric attacks language itself, suggesting that fateful words drive a poor soul into oblivion. To be sure, becoming part of a logic seeming to derive from the voice of the *other* reconstitutes the self's experience of maternal speech. Back to the body not getting enough from this mother, fixed by her discourse into a performance of sorts, the anorectic's stance is a psycho-somatic signifier pointing towards the mother who has failed the self. It is worth remembering, however, that the mother who fails is the internal object that the hysteric has constructed – reflecting the experience of the mother – but which is now part of the self's independent motivation to disable the internal father by succumbing to a mentally defective internal mother who craves a carrot a day, a child's body and a cartoon mentality to go with it all.

In Chapter 12 we shall return to aspects of this drive to return to childhood; but now we turn to the hysteric's penchant for showing the self.

Notes

1 This very important concept was coined by Clifford Scott (p. 333).
2 For a brilliant cultural analysis of hysteria in modern times, see Elaine Schowalter's book *Hystories* (1997).

Chapter 9

Showing off

Hysterical suffering, Freud believed, was a way of remembering the self's childhood. Symptoms were simply different ways of recalling the people and events of the past; histrionics a skilful means of portrayal.

Sometimes the body itself became the signifier of the other's effect on the self, indicating the nature of that original division when the body retained much of the psychic pain of rejection from the maternal real.

As discussed in previous chapters, the mother of the hysteric – either because of character or because of circumstance – cannot express a mother's erotic relation to her infant through breast-feeding and touch, and instead substitutes voice and performance, giving the child a scene of a mother's love, in which portrayal substitutes for embodied mothering. For some it means living inside maternal narrative as her internal object, taking one's place in her imagination, identifying with it, and enacting it before her eyes.

It is as if the mother says 'I shall enact a mother's love of her infant', giving the infant a role in her performance. It is not so difficult to see how the mother regards performance-as-the-thing-itself and why she may assert it powerfully, promoting the right of the maternal imaginary: to imagine the child is to be with the child. The popular phrases 'the inner child' and 'the child within' are apt descriptions of the hysteric's imagination. Later, if her child becomes hysteric then the child, too, will defend the imaginary with passion and aggression as it carries objects of love.

But the hysteric seeks to find the self in the other and comes to regard identification as the essential act of matriculation into the world. Everyone identifies with their mother, but normally the self uses aspects of the other to articulate its idiom, rather than the other way around, when the other is employed to articulate the object that is inside the other.

As the hysteric believes the core self is inside the mother, he or she becomes unusually concerned with inhabiting others, where the self is believed to reside, and where it is sought in order to materialise the other's desire.

We can easily see the strains of this kind of identification, especially if we appreciate that the hysteric is taking in a performance that is the mother's repudiated – yet partially realised – desire. Usually when we think of identification we imagine an object that can be identified with, that is somehow stable and clear.

Children go to films and emerge identified for a period of time with a hero or heroine, whom they portray and it is clear who is being presented.

As we shall discuss in the next chapter, those hysterics who become more seriously disturbed are caught up in the portrayal of a fragmented other. Either the mother or the father, or both, empty their internal lives through actings out into their children, who now become rather stunned witnesses. The parents' unconscious lives occupy the other, and the child may experience the other as an affliction.

A family law is established which licenses acting out as communication, a law that transforms inner states of mind into mad scenes that capture others. The self now *transformed into an event*, casts its internal objects into actual others, given roles in a drama only dimly apprehended. It can be highly exciting.

Freud clearly understood this aspect of hysterical theatre. In 'A note on the unconscious in psychoanalysis' (1912) he wrote that 'the mind of the hysterical patient is full of active yet unconscious ideas.' He continued:

> If she is executing the jerks and movements of her 'fits', she does not even consciously represent to herself the intended actions, and she may perceive those actions with the detached feelings of an onlooker. Nevertheless analysis will show that she was acting her part in the dramatic reproduction of some incident in her life.

(p. 262)

The hysteric does not 'represent to herself' the 'active yet unconscious ideas' in her 'full' mind, she acts them out in 'movements'. She divides herself between the fitful being caught up in her body-theatre and a 'detached . . . onlooker', a feature of the hysteric that Masud Khan[1] was to stress: the hysteric is *always* watching the self as theatre, or, as Freud put it, 'acting her part in the dramatic reproduction of some incident'.

Hysterical theatre is dream-like. It is as if the hysteric and his or her companion (including the analyst) are to believe that because hysterical enactment is a dream, it is authenticated by the deep meaning of dream life itself. For the hysteric, to be in the dream is to be inside the maternal unconscious, as dream experience recreates the sense of being inside the imaginative intelligence of the other. Hysterics' mothers and fathers are theatrical, casting the net of hysterical dream work into the family space. It can be deeply confusing.

A patient.

> It's hard to describe my parents, because in many many ways they were quite remarkable people, very accomplished, and 'high flyers'. They were both very powerful personalities and tempestuous and capable of the most extraordinary scenes. For example, it was not at all uncommon that at dinner they would begin discussing some topic that created differences between them – it could be just a political topic, for example – and they would soon be calling each other names. Mother would call father a 'penis head' and he would call her a

'stupid bitch' and I recall one time when she threw food at him across the table, actually catching my sister in its path. He jumped up and threw mashed potato at her, hitting her full square in the face, whereupon she threw her chair at him, and ran after him. They ran around the house, got down on all fours, and spit and cursed at each other. Then one or the other began laughing and soon they were roaring with laughter. On one occasion they returned to the table, apologised to all of us – and went on eating. That was what was so unbelievably strange. To my knowledge they never hurt each other, and they would return to a bizarre calm in which they acted as if nothing ever happened. My brothers and my sister and I were almost always completely transfixed by this, rather suspended in some kind of strange Disneyland ride. But I think it was also exciting, much like a roller coaster ride is exciting. We knew when it started that we were all in for a very mixed experience: partly paralysed, partly exhilarated, partly . . . proud? Proud, I think, because there was something so incredibly daring in them. I mean, they were doing things to one another that no one is supposed to do to anyone else, at least not in a civilised family. Although there were times when we were really freaked out we were also very protective of them and did not tell our relatives or anyone else, so far as I can recall.

Parents like this divest themselves of self holding and demand it of the family members, almost always the child witnesses. They use the group process as an alternative to the intrapsychic one, transforming self into an event that affects the group members. The child witness is usually silenced until adolescence, when he or she may in turn act out. Until then, the hysteric hides inside the good-boy or good-girl self as an innocent, all the while conceiving of objects derived from fragmented parental enactings.

The severely disturbed hysteric is populated by parental projective identifications, containing unprocessed fragments of the parents' unconscious, often warring with each other. The narcissistic character would aim to be oblivious to such outpourings; a schizoid to detach from it and study it; the borderline to find in its decompensating turbulence the affective embrace of the love object. The hysteric becomes the understudy who one day will take the stage.

European analysts often speak of the madness of the hysteric, referring to a certain type of bizarre behaviour which can move into a very particular type of activity, when vivid bizarre scenes are created in order to communicate the hysteric's inner life to the other. Although such hysterics may lose certain ego functions in doing so, it is a strange loss, because it derives from a kind of manic overcompensation, as they have precociously absorbed more of the object world than was good for them. Containing too many mad scenes and others within, they solve the problem of overcrowding by emptying fragments into the witness now possessed by them. In this way, hysteria is passed on from one generation to the next and is always catching. The madness of the bizarre internal world which contains the other's externalised internal objects is 'returned to sender'.

Not uncommonly, of course, the hysteric is unknowingly holding the mother's relation to *her* mother and father, or the father's relation to *his* parents. Indeed, one scene may be between the mother's mother and the father's father. The hysteric witness may contain many bizarrely crafted links.

The paralysis of the hysteric has much to do with that state of fear and excitement brought about by being the one acted upon, something which the hysteric uses in later life when he or she acts upon the other – including the analyst – to paralysing effect. Young clinicians are often intimidated into apology, reassurance or a type of empathy rather than analysis. They feel speechless and emptied, often experiencing in their countertransference the felt speechlessness and emptiness of the child blown away by parental enactment.[2]

But hysterical acting out is not only aimed at reversing their fortune, for – in analysis especially – they are also asking if anyone can make sense of this mess. Furthermore, containing such fragments does at times lead to compassion for the parents, and promotes an empathic skill of sorts, as the hysteric perceives the parents' use of the family space as a holding environment to contain their inner world. As the parents often return to ordinary living after such scenes, making reparation and expressing sorrow, some hysterics have a sense of having held the vulnerable aspects of their parents' selves.

In the art of showing off, of putting into forms of relational performance aspects of one's inner life, the hysteric makes himself or herself available for a type of knowing, just as he or she has seen aspects of the parents' internal worlds from the way they have openly enacted them.

Masud Khan (1983b) writes of a patient called 'Judy' in 'None can speak his/her folly': 'she exploited her environment negatively, to her disadvantage as a person. It was very much like a caricature of her mother's character' (p. 60). The hysteric sustains identifications by caricature of self and others – a form of cancellation by parody that reveals a type of despair expressed through self-debasement.

Self caricature (in the form of bizarre actings out) is unconsciously intended to elicit a firm analytical response aimed at deconstructing the caricature. The hysteric challenges the other to end the madness by apprehending the caricature, but the resolution of the madness is not so much to analyse all the meanings of the contained, but to analyse the process.

There is no question that this puts the analyst in what seems to be a dire struggle between the mad family and sanity. Indeed, as the hysteric's aim is to re-project the madness into the analyst – i.e. to pass it along – the analyst's challenge of the system feels initially as if he or she is refusing to hold the patient.

The analyst must also learn to deal with what we might think of as the hysterical picaresque. Just as family scenes unfolded in an odyssey through childhood, the hysteric finds in the natural unfolding of life's events another skeleton to be exploited for the intense evacuations of self and other into the natural event. A holiday, a visit from a friend, a shopping trip, a wedding: any of these may become opportunities for distorted and crazy occasions. The hysteric will then often recount these mad scenes as if reading from *Moll Flanders*: these free associations are like picaresque episodes, sustaining more than communicating unconscious madness. We can see this in Breuer and Freud's *Studies on Hysteria* – with Emmy, for example – where for a while he saw his task as one of 'erasing' from mind her presentation of a disturbing scene. Interestingly, Freud may have been trying to create a truly blank screen when in fact there was 'clutter', as Khan (1983b) says of Judy.

Anticipating a visit from Judy – who has been away for several years – Khan says, 'I cannot expect her to free associate or speak her madness, because she would not know how to speak – what, how, to whom!' (p. 73). No one knew how to speak. Part of the 'show and tell' of the hysteric is the unconscious representation of the confused child watching it all. Hysterical mad scenes are highly overdetermined events in which this child self is watching a scene – sometimes begging for understanding – amidst a bizarre occasion that the hysteric has set in motion.

Symptoms are held scenes, events contained in the self, to which the hysteric still bears witness in a dissociated way. In more severe hysterias the symptom is released into the group, now and then to be returned to the self as symptom.

Psychotic decompensation in the hysteric is peculiar. He or she hallucinates or fosters delusions, but still remains witness to the psychosis, much as he or she witnessed family madness. Only now the hysteric witnesses the unconscious enacted in this way.

These moments – and the non-psychotic scenes – are like thing presentations, the performing of the unforgettable image not transformed into a word presentation, that would echo and change it. Is the conversion symptom, especially the one guided by the word, an attempted transformation into word presentation? Is the use of the body as sign, whether enervated or cut up, a return to the body from which a symbolising self was meant to emerge? Is the body symptom therefore a sign of hope, a step toward the symbolic that has body integrity, authorised from within?

The hysteric symptom is not simply self containment but possibly self symbolisation: especially the creation of a secret not so *easily* discussed, much less figured. The search is to be a mystery, yes, to be able to create secrets – the unconscious – of one's own and not the other, which deserves time and the patient presence of the other to figure.

Freud realised as early as *Studies* (Breuer and Freud, 1893) that his patients were not telling him the full story. Less aware of the transference than he was eventually to become, he could not see the patient's investment in maintaining the horrors of the visual and of playing down the full verbal disclosure. For in sustaining the image in opposition to speech, the hysteric sequestered the first order of communication with the primary object: the visual exchange with the other. In her maddening clowning as an adult, the hysteric remembers the mother's visual reflections of infancy, of a mother aiming to crack up her baby.

In preferring the imaginary to the symbolic order, or in sustaining visual impact over verbal communication, the hysteric preserves his or her investment in the maternal order to the comparative exclusion of the paternal order. An image is worth a thousand scenes. An enactment is open to any interpretation. Two souls can go wild with speculations and overlapping desires. A fully told story, however, is repeatable and can be examined. Polysemous words are also telling in a way that the image is not. If you slip and choose the wrong word, it cannot be erased: it has been spoken. So the hysteric will choose the performative over the narrative, with narrative inseparable from its performative intentions. When speaking, the hysteric is always acting upon the other, like a lyric poem acting in the world of conventional prose.

The performances are not superficial. It is a showing by a relocating evocation. What the hysteric brings up in his or her performance always evokes something inside the gathered witnesses and sponsors internal imaginings, where he or she is dispersed through the other's imaginary.

When the psychoanalyst supports the supremacy of the spoken word over the act, it facilitates the patient's matriculation in the paternal order. This transformation is mirrored in the core psychoanalytic experience when the patient recollects the dream. Remembering the night's dream is to bring the imaginary order into a new place as the communications of infant and mother are brought into the space of self and father. Freud insists that the remembered dream – a token of the maternal order – be subjected to free association, in which differing images are broken down and words hidden within them are revealed.

But this transformation is not part of the dream work itself. It is the work of psychoanalysis and the analytical interpreter who penetrates the dream and breaks it down. Most patients feel this as a type of violence. The dream is the thing-itself, a pure ego experience, a revelation that should be allowed to stand untouched and admired, a token of the infant–mother supremacy. But Freud would have none of it and despatched this infantile bond with paternal admonition bordering on contempt.

Through free association, however, Freud joined the maternal and the paternal orders. The patient allowed simply to speak what came to mind seemed almost a maternal defiance of the demands to get to the truth; if so, then it only borrowed from the psychic reality that no truth could ever be imposed, but rather had to be created. During such reveries the psychoanalyst would be in an evenly suspended state of mind – not concentrating on anything, not remembering anything, not reflecting on anything – until such time as a connecting thread in the material became apparent, which he or she would then interpret. The patient and analyst might conjure the medium of mother and small child – a world of overlapping reveries – but in this case the father would intervene with his discovery of important communications, lucid lessons and the patient's hidden conflicts. All along, of course, this simply mirrored the self's conviction that anything found by the father was a truth searching for its repressions in the comforting arms of the maternal universe.

To Korfman, Freud's wish was that the 'power of the theoretical should dominate the myth' (1980: 79), where 'myth' suggests the omnipotence of the mother, a pre-eminence that links her function with death (something which,

Freud argues, we all regard as personally impossible). The sleuth-like dream interpreter walks in the footsteps of the father who would convert the maternal order (image and 'myth') to the paternal order (word and 'truth').

Interestingly, Korfman cites Freud's recollection in the dream book of his mother's first lesson. The mother tells her 6-year-old son that we are all made of earth and shall return to earth. When she meets with his scepticism, she rubs her hands together to show him her epidermis. 'My astonishment at this ocular demonstration knew no bounds and I acquiesced in the belief which I was later to hear expressed in the words: *"Du bist der Natur einen Tod schuldig"*' (Dreams: 205). Korfman (1980) does not comment on Freud's formal transformation of this event and as such does not catch how Freud moves from the maternal to the paternal order in the space of one sentence. His affect exists in the astonishments created by maternal 'ocular demonstration' – the world of maternal image-making which we have been discussing – but as soon as he can, Freud moves from the image to the word, and the sentence concludes with the memory of a phrase which displaces the oneiric. Thus the man who teaches us how dream imagery must be supplanted by verbal comprehension indicates in his own dream book the recollection of transforming maternal imagery into verbal sense; or, in the Lacanian lexicon, how the child must move the maternal imaginary into the paternal symbolic discourse.

It has often been said that Freud did not comprehend the child's relation to the mother nearly as well as he understood the functions of the father. So, it is touching and more than sad when we look back on the concluding paragraph of his footnote on Emmy. 'It was not for another quarter of a century that I once more had news of Frau Emmy' he tells us (1893: 105), before mentioning that her elder daughter had approached him for a report on her mother's mental condition. The daughter, now a doctor, together with her sibling, had been disowned by Emmy and was now proceeding to 'take legal proceedings against her mother, whom she represented as a cruel and ruthless tyrant'. Who knows how matters would have fared had Freud understood that each hysteric feels the tyranny of the mother's over-appropriation of the self.

Our consideration of the hysteric is now at a transitional point, between the ordinary and the malignant forms. In the less disturbed hysteric, where we may imagine a more contained mother and father, the child hysteric enacts the maternal object of desire – and moves on to the father as well – in the presence of the parent, who concurs with the representation. The self becomes unusually skilled in identifying and representing the imagined other's desire and part of this imagining is the performance of the object in the presence of the other.

Importantly, however, this hysteric does not have a mother inflicting herself upon the other – indeed, rather the opposite: the mother has receded into herself, especially insofar as her erotic objects are concerned. She has to be pursued. She has to be fathomed. It is necessary to join her auto-erotic reveries through a seance of one's own auto-erotisms. What one performs for her is the materialisation of a secret. Its manifestation is the smile crossing the silent face.

The malignant hysteric faces an opposing problem. Often the mother and father violently empty their inner lives – especially their sexual states of mind – into the children, who then become containers of vividly unforgettable scenes. The mother and father transform themselves into events and capture the children as audiences.

If the contents of the ascetic and malignant representations are both erotic, the ways of expressing them are wildly different. In the ascetic stance the hysteric acts out a scene of obvious auto-erotic reference in the presence of the other. It is puzzling. Odd. But not inflictual. In the malignant stance the self empties its inner scenes into the other, who becomes transfixed and traumatised by the other's use of them as parts of the performance.

We cannot leave this chapter on showing off the self without returning to the body and its drives. Let us recall the child who opens his or her legs and displays the genital to the mother: remember that the hysterical mother cannot find wording for this showing. Whether she affects a stony silence, which we speculate is the antecedent of the ascetic solution, or whether she giggles or laughs in a manic and excited way, which may bias the child to the precocious form of hysteria, her words do not enter the child's body to become part of the body's memory of this early showing of sexuality.

Becoming an event, where the self is a kind of visual order overwhelming the verbal dimension, which it exploits to its own scene-making intentions, the hysteric has de-genitalised the early showing and spread it through the entire body, which is now shown in all its indiscriminate forms. As we shall discuss later when considering certain patients in some depth, this showing turns all the body parts into erotic agents, each a showing of the genital, but so diffused that although the self is immolated in sexuality, this is not finally a genital offering. What word could the witness to this event put to the occasion? What could one say?

The absence of maternal containment of the child's exhibitionistic sexuality, of his or her showing off of the genital – a containment that must be put into words – reveals itself in the performative violation of the function of words, now used as agents of action, and not as means of symbolically processing the unconscious contents.

Wording sexuality puts the self's body into language; hence the symbolic order. Displacing the sexual into the non-sexual or anti-sexual wordings – 'oh, you are a good boy', or 'that's nasty' – either fails to move the sexual into language or encumbers the body with its desire. The hysteric's conversion of sexual desire into the body is not a new-found mode of action on the part of the hysteric; rather, it is the route for the unwording of desire which is to be left to the body suffering from it. The psychoanalytic cure is not simply to put thoughts into words, but more pertinently, to allow the subject's desire to find its own words – thereby symbolically restoring in the transference the maternal function of wording the self's body. However important the detective discovery of the precise contents of the repressed ideas might be – here, the work of the father looking for the hidden – the form of wording itself, of putting one's states of mind into words which shape them, is the work of the maternal order. In so many ways the hysterical mother is gifted at wording, but in her ambivalence over her own sexuality, she either refuses, or displaces, or shatters her child's presentation of the sexual body for its wording. Psychoanalytical work recuperates that wording and moves the hysteric from angry and evacuative performances of the sexual to wording it in a symbolic order that allows the self to repossess the body and its desire.

Freud comprehended (unconsciously, at the very least) that hysterical attacks bear something of the history of the mother and the child, because in discussing 'the motor phenomena of hysterical attacks' in 'The preliminary communication' of *Studies on Hysteria*, he and Breuer wrote that such attacks

> can be interpreted partly as universal forms of reaction appropriate to the affect accompanying the memory (such as kicking about and waving the arms and legs, which even young babies do), partly as a direct expression of these memories.
>
> (p. 15)

Evoking the baby's body points us unconsciously back to the earliest forms of body expression and, of course, to the first relation. In another place, at another time, Freud would describe the mother's relation to her infant as in all respects a love relation, with the infant the mother's lover. By likening the hysteric's attacks to the infant's flailing body, Freud cannily linked the original trauma to the mother. However, my view is that, because he could not identify (and therefore could not solve) this trauma, he understood it as actual sexual abuse by men, and subsequently as fantasies. If we take the original trauma to be, ironically enough, a failed seduction where the mother cannot word either the 'waving . . . arms and legs' or the displayed genitals, then the only way in which the infant can rescue the self from this absence of sensorial confirmation and verbal transformation of the self's sexuality is to resort to fantasy. The abuse conundrum – did it really happen, or is it imagined? – is in this respect a dual memory, a link, between a happening that did not occur except in fantasy, which was essential to repair the damage of the non-event.

Mother and child who are left to show off only to one another have at least been to a theatre together. On the stage of the genital show – in early infancy – child shows mother his or her genital and mother shows child that she does not have words for that part of the body. They remain stuck in a showing that displaces the shown, that throws the genital signifier into objects and events that are meant to lose it. Maternal guilt may drive increasingly artful showings and tellings to the child, desperate to recuperate something lost, thereby repeating the form of loss in the very work, ironically, of the presumed recuperation. 'Come and look at this!' and 'Sit down, I have a story to tell you!' become excitements of the mother conveyed to the excited child, thrills running through the body brought about by narrative and performances, but the wording bears the loss of desire.

It is to further discussion of this tragic form of theatre that we now turn.

Notes

1   See 'Grudge and the hysteric', in *Hidden Selves* (Khan, 1983).
2   See my 'The psychoanalyst and the hysteric', in *The Shadow of the Object* (Bollas, 1985).

Chapter 10

Self as theatre

It is common to portray an hysteric as theatrical without giving it much further thought. It seems an apt description of a particular neurotic style, as it quickly brings to mind the antics of a certain sort of person – the scatterbrained woman being a typical stereotype.

One patient, for example, typically collided with her fellow citizens, such as the day she commented on a fellow commuter's shoes, and whilst moving to touch the admired objects provoked an involuntary recoil from the shoe-wearer, who spilled her bag of shopping on to the floor. This inspired another passenger to quickly drop to the floor of the Underground carriage in order to pick up the fallen objects. However, his good intentions were momentarily thwarted by the patient, who also dropped to the floor only to bump into him. In the next few seconds several other passengers came to the aid of the jostling threesome and as the folly continued it took several minutes for the passengers to return to their ordinary lives.

However, another stereotype exists in male culture: that of the homosexual man who appears camply dramatic, provoking looks of amused astonishment from those surrounding him. A patient, for example, loved to wear women's hats, which he knew turned heads. Onlookers would be greeted by an amused expression on his face that might be translated as 'I know, isn't this absolutely outrageous, but what are we to make of this nonsense?', a beguiling and friendly self-mockery that further confused the other, who would often say something like 'A special occasion?' or 'That must be fun', verging on an unexpected speaking engagement with the patient, which threw them into a type of intimacy. One day, for example, he elicited this response from a greengrocer, who said he thought all men should wear such hats, only to find that the patient then constructed a hat out of some greens, which he invited the grocer to wear, which he did – immediately and awkwardly – in turn bringing howls of delight from passers-by, who made enquiries and offered further suggestions. Undoubtedly, the greengrocer has never forgotten this event, even if he is unsure of what overcame him in that moment.

It is an oddity of the hysteric that he or she senses and delivers the other's perception of the stereotype, fulfilling the role of the scatterbrain or the camp self. But it is a skill evolved from countless acts of fulfilling the imagined object of the other's desire, in which the true self is suspended whilst a stand-in takes its place. We can see the aggressive features of this enactment; indeed, the above scenes express a type of violation. But it is a comic rather than tragic enactment. Ordinarily, the topsy-turvy world will return to normal in the end, and mayhem will have been seen to be the work of a slightly daffy woman or man, who will genially accept responsibility for having brought about disruption.

In the art of transforming the self into an event the hysteric sets the stage for the personification of absent others, even enlisting passers-by to perform unknown roles in the unfolding drama. This creates a special mood, composed of surprise, uncertain expectation and anxiety, as it is not clear how this living theatre – or agitprop – will turn out. Who will appear? Who is being called up? And in what company?

Hysterical theatre is always something of a seance, as ghosts of the past are brought into some strange light and the hysteric feels himself or herself to be something of a medium for the transition of the absents into a type of materialisation. This lends itself to a sense of the self as sacrificial host, but one who is even expert. There is true dramatic skill involved in the continuous evocation of parts of the mother, or parts of the father, or a brother, or a long since completed family event which only lives on in its theatrical rendering.

We know that the hysterical skill evolves out of a conviction that one's apparent self is to be found in the maternal narrative and performance. As the mother tells the child about herself and her child, or as she acts out the character of this relationship, she hints who this child is to her. As this is not a secure identity, however, the child becomes accustomed to sensing that his or her fate as the maternal internal object will vary according to her moods, her states of mind and especially her sexual conflicts. An uplifting aspect of this state of affairs is the sense of one's considerable significance to the mother's inner life, even if this is a conflicted existence. One can see the mother struggling with her child, either verbally by openly considering her points of view in the presence of her child – a type of sharing – or by performatively indicating her own many views of the child even in the course of a few minutes.

Helen, for example, recalled the following moment as typical of her mother.

> In the morning mother would *be* a kind of chanticleer stirring us from our slumber and marshalling us to the kitchen for the family breakfast. We all had pet names. My brother was called 'goat' and I was called 'kika' and she would talk to us with great affection, but also casting us into roles before we were fully awake. So she would say to my brother 'So where has goat been in the night? With the woolly footballies and the knobbly knockabouts . . .' and she would go on in language which we understood because she had this amazing knack of giving us an affectionate private language for ourselves and others, and she was rather like a whirlwind of fun and organisation in the morning. But as soon as we left for school – as any of us would see when we stayed home for one reason or another – she would dramatically collapse, her voice would drop an octave, she would visibly change in her face from cheerfulness

to something like deep suffering, and then she would stare at us and say with searching gaze 'So Helen . . . so my little Helen . . . what do you think of it all . . . um?' I don't know what I said when I was young, but later when this would go on and I would say something she would nod knowingly as if she already had thought out what I was saying, so it was always as if I was somehow still living inside her. When I was an adolescent this would annoy me no end and she would get cross and accuse me of being an ungrateful child, which was true to some extent, and I would always feel guilty because she was, in her own way, deeply loving. And back to the day, after a period of searching, she would suddenly change into another self, then another self, and by the end of the day she had been in so many places, and I had been so many different Helens, that it was like watching a film about one's life directed by some amazing life force.

Importantly, the mother provides the child with multiplicity. There are many selves and many others in this theatre and one can see fragments of who one is to the mother at any moment in time. The set pieces, following one another in the course of an ordinary day, are clear and symbolically cohesive. So if Helen is 'kika' in the morning – a word that captures her spirit as a kind of good kicker – and valued as something of an athletic presence, she may be Helen the wise as soon as the table is cleared, followed by Helen the numbskull by late morning, followed by the figures who cross the mother's mind, expressed in her voice-over of lived experience, performed before her daughter. The coherence of these set pieces allows the child to enter any particular one of them upon further reflection and to find certain unconscious riches as the mother conveys the shades of unconscious meanings through her narrations.

Before considering the problems this kind of mothering may sponsor, it is important to see its accomplishments. This mother constantly transforms the everyday into theatre. She animates her family, and gives them secure places and roles in a dynamic interplay of unconscious elements that amounts to a kind of sharing-out of the maternal unconscious. These children are continuously reborn through maternal transformation and their mothers are often valued for their uncanny skill in perceiving something of the child's idiom, characterising it, and giving it a part in a set-piece drama that has as many variations as there are days in a lifetime.

Indeed, if we see this process as generative, we can see how some hysterics indicate a history of participation in forms of self–other interaction based on quite uncanny unconscious communications. Harold, for example, recalls the richness of his mother's stories: her accounts of her parents' lives, of her childhood, of her many friends, and of her many accomplishments. Even though he and his brothers knew many of these stories quite well they still enjoyed hearing them narrated again and again. His mother was a very passionate and emotional woman, whose own narrations would move her to fury, pensive reflectiveness, or tears. These were rather spellbinding moments. Harold's father, although sometimes critical of the mother for going on a bit, also seemed to love her for her deep feelings, her remarkable memory, and her astonishing skill in bringing people and events to life. Harold also recalls how she would tell him stories about himself. As he went to school, to a sports event, to visit a friend, or for a bike ride she would narrate his roles. 'Now when you see your teacher, don't get caught up in being a rival with your friend Ted for her affection. You are strong and independent and you have your own future, so just listen to her and don't . . .'. In early adolescence, he was aware of how her imaginings were often quite wrong, but he did not feel angry with her. Indeed, not only did he find these stories pleasurable and entertaining, but he also understood them to be expressions of her commitment and love, and he did not want to disabuse her of her right to possess him in this way. It was no 'skin off [his] nose' if she was wrong. Occasionally, he was surprised at how prophetic her stories were – although at first he would shrug to himself and reckon she was quite out of it, later her notion of what was in him would prove to be a reality. Importantly, she did not take offence when he was kidding her by giving his views on what was preoccupying her. They would engage in something like mutual narrating of the other's true state of mind. Looking back, he felt he had learned a great deal about people through this form of play – about how to get inside the other through active imagination, how to share the other's inner life.

If Harold's story is typical of the child who is not disposed to become an hysteric by maternal hysteria, indeed who even gains comprehension and appreciation of life and others through it, then the flip side is the child who gets caught up in the maternal world by identifying with her internal representations, then enacting these differing selves in her presence. By extension, however, this also means evolving a capacity to get inside any other, not only to identify oneself as the other's internal object and then to enact it, but further to identify with all findable internal objects and to represent them to the other. These children have managed to cultivate a type of empathic skill in which they get inside the other and act the other out. This is, of course, unconscious. It is driven by anxiety about being left out in the cold unless one can find the self inside the other, and in the best of times a type of warmth is found in playing oneself to the other, a form of mirroring in which the child reflects the mother's internal objects.

In the more complex hysterias a child is caught up in maternal memory, unknowingly acting out parts of the mother's differing child selves in her own history, as well as parts of the mother's mother's personality and the mother's father's personality, in densely complex rememberings. One patient recalls his mother's frequent description of his likeness to her father. He was gentle and pensive, and one day he would smoke a pipe like her father. She shared this story with her mother, who also adopted it, and the grandmother would sing a song – 'Oh my papa' – which was not simply a type of dedicated memory to her long since dead husband, but a fusion of her grandson with his grandfather. It was not until this person was an adult that, in the course of his analysis, he realised that for significant periods in his childhood he *was* this grandfather, insofar as his mother and grandmother were concerned, and, further, that he sought to identify with him.

It is not too difficult to see that when hysterics become psychotic they often portray themselves through a bewildering array of characters. That they may hallucinate persons, or that they may shift enacted identifications with alarming and bizarre speed, should not earn them a diagnosis of schizophrenia; they are not projectively identifying split-off parts of the mind (as in schizophrenia) but instead collecting into one space all the characters with whom they have been identified throughout their life. As the self is a medium for the transportation of the other's objects, hysterics can enter strangely altered states of consciousness in which they seem to be inhabited and spoken through, followed by a period of exhaustion, stricken by the event of transportation. Even a non-psychotic hysteric, such as Helen's mother, would often collapse in exhaustion after a period of carrying and portraying something. 'Okay . . . enough of that . . . enough of that', she would say, with a sweep of the hand, and occasionally with a laugh, springing out of whatever had been inhabiting her mind and preoccupying her actions.

Children of hysterics, however, are usually more than good, quiet, spellbound audiences. In the economy of being the good boy or the good girl, the child seen but not heard – certainly not interruptively so – is especially valued as a kind of mirror child, who discovers that absence of response is taken to be appreciation of the mother's desire. This may be a saving grace, however, as the witnesses to maternal performance are also often momentarily paralysed by the sheer power of the performance. Robert:

> When mom would embark on one of her accounts of an event, no one would interrupt her, and she would demand a kind of fiercely concentrated attention. If you looked the other way, or seemed restless, or worse, bored, she would fly into a fury. Once she chased me around the house because I made a face when she was telling a story about what the school bus driver had indicated to her about her driving.

Robert recalls feeling frozen by both the power and the intensity of his mother's stories. Fortunately, there were many pleasant aspects to her character in her non-hysterical states, but when she launched into one of her tellings, everyone pretty well dropped whatever they were doing and stood at attention. He believes that the more impulsive she was, the more stiff and controlled he became, but at the time of his analysis, when he was considering this part of his life, he was more concerned with sudden eruptions within himself of his mother's way of being. Having been unusually good and dutiful throughout his adolescence and into his twenties, he found that in his early thirties he was given to uncharacteristic outbursts of exhibitionistic storytelling in which he got 'unbelievably involved' in narrating a story. He was surprised to discover that when describing an ordinary event he would soon embellish it and the story would take on a life of its own. It would carry him away and soon he would be mixing fact with fiction in a narrative panoply that was deeply satisfying. This occurred after marriage and the birth of his second child, and he was aware that it flowered in the context of his telling stories of his work life to his wife and children. When he saw that he was paralysing the family – they all seemed to stop breathing when he was telling an event – he decided he was acting like his mother and sought psychoanalysis.

It is not uncommon for a person to fight with his or her own hysteria in this way. Robert was not at ease with his acting out and in fighting it off he felt as if he were deliberately refusing an identification with his mother. On the other hand, he felt that his acting out self was an important part of him, that he had held it in abeyance all these years whilst being a good boy, and he struggled with the satisfactions it yielded.

Marilyn found herself in a different situation. Although she found her mother's performance anxiety provoking, she also felt a desperate need to be of true interest to her mother, whom she experienced as spilling herself out so often that she seemed to have trouble remembering who people were. For example, in a family of three children, Marilyn's mother was always mixing up the children's names, and frequently Marilyn would hear her name announced last amongst the three. The mother would often convert it into a joke, however, by then naming one or more of the family pets, mocking her inability to keep an accurate name in mind at any one time. Marilyn did discern the mother's favourite version of Marilyn, and she was determined to be this perfect little girl as frequently as possible. One of the gratifying aspects of this was that she could hear the mother remember her good deeds. She gained access to her mother's internal world by acting out a favourite part, which she then could hear recounted in future stories. This was in stark contrast to one of her sisters, who refused to collaborate with the mother and embarked on what was to be a long history of deviant defiance of parental authority. When the mother narrated the important moments of family life that day or that week the naughty sister was never mentioned. It was as if she did not exist.

In Marilyn's mother, then, there seemed to be vivid, rather jumbled stories of the members of the family, as long as they were collaborative with the mother. So she would tell the story of one child going with her to the store and what happened there, or another child going to the hairdresser's, but she negated the unwanted, which existed as the unnarrated object. This drove a wish in Marilyn to exist in some meaningful way in her mother's discourse by identifying with the internal object that lived in her name, presenting it to the mother as often as possible. She felt her mother would recall her, but it was a recollection supplied by the belief that her mother was constantly losing her internal objects through her narratives.

Our discussion of hysteria has repeatedly focused on how the mother bears the imaginary child in her narrative and indicates a relation through performance, a link forged between the narrative and the performative act. But we have not distinguished the psychic significance of that difference which is suggested by the balance between the two – between the mother who narrates the child to himself or herself and the mother who shows the child who he is to himself, or who she is to herself. Joel's account is useful.

My mother was a *phenom*. She loved to talk and talk and talk and she was very interesting. And my sister and I were almost always amused by the amazing ramblings and perambulations of her interests, from opera to politics, and from what the neighbours did to what was in the *TLS*: it was a kind of cornucopia. But often, too often for all of us, she would seem frustrated by the limitations of narrative and she would jump up and show us what she was talking about. So if she was talking about a moment in *Electra* she jumped up and acted out *Electra*, or if she saw two neighbours having a dispute she acted both of them out in front of us. It's very hard to say what upset us about this, because as I recall it now, there is something almost touching and sweet about her. But it did make us anxious as I think we never quite knew to what limits she would take her dramatics. Further, when we were in a public place there were times when she would insist upon showing us something instead of just telling us, and by the time we were in our twenties, I remember too often that one of us would say 'Mom, sit down, and just tell us' or we would see that she was just about to leap to her feet to show us and we would say to her 'Mom, now don't get up . . . just stay put and tell us.' There were a few times, fortunately only a few, when she would feel deeply hurt by our response. There would be a puzzled look on her face, as if we were taking from her an important part of herself. And she would burst into hot angry tears and run from the room and lock herself in the other room. We would feel absolutely awful.

Joel's recollection is of his and his sister's resistance to a transformation from the narrative to the theatrical order, from simply telling an event to showing it. What might the nature of the anxiety surrounding the transition be? What is there in the movement from telling to showing that he found so distressing?

Might it be the transition from the symbolic to the imaginary order, from the world of words alone, to the scene itself? If so, then what the mother remembers and what the child fears is regression from the verbal to the imaginary, or, as Freud discussed it, from the word presentational to the thing presentational. The mother would then not simply be showing something as opposed to telling something, but would transform herself from a teller to a shower, or from the word to the image. It was the sight of the mother showing that plunged Joel and his sister into anxiety, because once she was on her feet portraying a scene in front of the children, she linked herself up to the children's earliest sense of vital evidence: that the truth comes through what you see, not what you conceptualise or what you hear. Seeing is believing.

This somewhat primitive notion of the truthful has important bases in psychic development. Why should someone believe that the truth comes with sight? Perhaps the evidence that generates this conviction is the inner sight we have of our dreams, where the most important truths of our unconscious reality are brought to our attention through vivid picturings – picturings that we do not witness from some remove, but of which we are an active part, sometimes to our great fright, occasionally to our deep pleasure. The sight of the mother who becomes a theatre of the other before our very eyes plays upon important unconscious memories not only of the convincing effect of the dream upon our selves, but of that link in the unconscious between the dream and the mother. As we return to a foetal state upon sleep, as we regress to a more infant-like form of mentation, we move back in time to the moments when we nestled against the mother, enwrapped in her body, enfolded in her arms and her voice. As discussed in the previous chapter, the sense we have as infants of being partly present inside a seemingly magical universe that transforms us is repeatedly remembered in dream experience, which in this respect recollects the nature of being with the mother.[1]

When Joel's mother jumped up to show her children what she was thinking, she may well have drawn upon her unconscious conviction that truth can only be conveyed by bringing others into her theatre to see in order to believe. For Joel the mother's transformation was a devolution back to the experience of being inside the earliest form of maternal process: of bringing the world to the self through its pictorial, sensorial and acoustic acuity. Words were a long way off. Sight and sound were right there at the beginning.

Freud understood hysterical theatre – which he called 'hysterical attacks' – as the enactment of a repressed sexual fantasy. A heretofore repressed sexual idea returns to a type of consciousness in the form of an enactment, with the patient acting out the fantasy, often in reverse order of its proper imagining. In 'Some general remarks on hysterical attacks' (1909a) Freud gives a short description of how this occurs:

> Supposing, for instance, that a hysterical woman has a phantasy of seduction in which she is sitting reading in a park with her skirt slightly lifted so that her foot is visible; a gentleman approaches and speaks to her; they then go somewhere and make love to one another. This phantasy is acted out in the attack by her beginning with the convulsive stage, which corresponds to the coitus, by her then getting up, going into another room, sitting down and reading and presently answering an imaginary remark addressed to her.
>
> (p. 231)

Freud sees such attacks, therefore, 'as nothing else but phantasies translated into the motor sphere' (p. 229), but because these are auto-erotic scenes put into theatre, and because all auto-erotic fantasy involves the self in an imaginary bisexuality (portraying both sexes), such enactments are accomplished 'through *multiple identification*' (p. 230).

Let us return, then, to our earlier discussion of the mother's narrative and performative externalisation of her erotic life before her child, one that primarily substitutes for her inability erotically to engage her infant's body. As argued, she shows enough of where her erotic life takes place to lure the child into a more intensive effort to find one's self inside the maternal theatre, where the self is – or is imagined to be – erotically welcomed. As repression is an erotic activity, and as the work of absence, according to Freud (1909a), is based on the loss of consciousness in orgasm, the maternal withdrawal of obvious erotic interest in the child is interpreted by the child's unconscious as an erotised absence, but one which suggests the very opposite – an overflowing, overwhelming erotic investment in the infant that must be repressed, lest all should be overcome.

When the hysteric transforms himself or herself into an event, externalising maternal performative-narrative, he or she does so as a form of erotic theatre, even if the specific contents of the mayhem seemingly have nothing to do with sexuality. For example, one performance may involve the person 'drawing back the arms convulsively till the hands meet over the spinal column', which would appear to be anything but erotic, but this example from Freud's cases could express an embrace transformed into its opposite. He then wonders if 'the well-known *arc de cercle* which occurs during attacks in major hysteria is nothing else than an energetic repudiation like this, through antagonistic innervation, of a posture of the body that is suitable for sexual intercourse' (1909a: 230).

These 'attacks' or 'theatrical enactments' are moments when the self chooses to devolve the customary representations of its singularity – suggesting a unified being who is in firm narrative grip of his or her inner life – in favour of the self as an event composed of a group of differing parts engaged in combat at least with each other and probably with others from their world. Sexuality is in the scene-making itself, in the work of visible representation. Here the inner world of erotic imagining and the actual world of unforgettable scenes are joined, as they were in the hysteric's relation to the mother, where both mother and child desisted from overt specific celebrations of their erotic relationship in favour of sequestration to masturbatory excitements and wonderfully inventive substitute representations in the actual world, where sexuality would remain disguised as the erotics of scene- making, regardless of the contents of the represented.

Children who become hysterics in adult life, given to 'attacks' or 'theatrical enactments', have been transformed by mothers who empty themselves into the group – primarily the family, but also friends at work and social groups. A process of transmission is suggested: instinctual states and their fantasies held in the body self will be transformed into the non-sexual event, but delivered in such a way as to transmit states of excitation to the other in the group, so that what was inside one self is now inside several different selves, none of which has sufficient presence of mind (or authority, perhaps) to recombine the erotic into a narrative capable of ending the attack. It is highly unlikely that a child in such a situation could say to the mother, 'When you are throwing the pans on to the floor and kicking them about, screaming at the top of your lungs, you are representing your wish to be thrown down on the ground by a forceful other and penetrated so that you can scream in delight', although at differing times and in differing ways psycho-analysts do attempt such interpretations.

When the self becomes an event startling the eyes of the other it illustrates the self possessed by the primal scene, driven into mad gestures that seem the violent intercourse of the self's parts. Driven to distraction by the imagined scene of parental intercourse, the hysteric tries to re-enter innocence through the shocked gaze of the other, who for a moment is an innocent in the presence of something happening beyond the witness's knowledge. In a flash, hysterics projectively identify themselves into the other, bathing in innocence. Yet the need to know, to evade exclusion by the parental couple from their power, compels the hysteric to 'face' the primal scene, the quintessential conundrum that evokes the self's need to know. So the hysteric explores this scene by appropriative identification, omnisciently enacting it so that it can be incorporated (not internalised) into the self. It is the bite of the apple, not the search for knowledge.

The frozen singularity of the ascetic hysteric – like Lot's wife – is the sign of the self paralysed by the sight of fucking. Although the ascetic hysteric is obviously less overtly theatrical than the precocious hysteric, he or she incorporates into his or her bodily being the annulments of the primal scene. One sees in the anorectic above all the ascetic self's dramatic effectiveness. As this self wastes away, the body is relentlessly reduced to signify only death-at-the-doorstep. Life has been taken from the body and now is to be found only in the agitated surrounding community (parents, friends, doctors), who become a mockery of the primal scene. For all their collective intercourses, the community cannot conceive of a way to stop the anorectic's death drive, ultimately a chilling attack on others as useless fuckers.

Hysterical theatre is always polymorphous as the self releases its sexual history in the devolution to becoming an event. Oral, anal, urethral, phallic, as well as visual, auditory and kinaesthetic component instincts now have momentary places on centre stage, shown off to the object world, in what can become a deeply disturbing regression to early sexual representations. We are now bordering on what is termed the 'malignant hysteric' and it is to this most demanding of all patients that we turn next.

Note

1   For further discussion of this topic please see my 'Origins of the therapeutic alliance', in *The Mystery of Things* (Bollas, 1999).

Chapter 11

The malignant hysteric

There is unlikely to be a clinic in Europe which is not visited every so often by what some of its staff will call a 'malignant hysteric', something of an awesome figure in the psychoanalytical world. Yet when they do materialise, one sees why analysts speak in rather hushed tones and with some trepidation, because these are remarkably disturbing people. If one looks through the analytical literature, however, there are very few references to these people who are talked of so much and whose appearances are so memorable. So what is a malignant hysteric?

It was Michael Balint who distinguished between 'benign' and 'malignant' forms of regression in analysis. Patients who gradually abandon higher-level functioning in the course of the natural regressions that occur through transference experiencing are those for whom the experience is likely to be benign. Even if they discover deeply meaningful self experiences and encounter painful but essential news about the self, and discover through transference dependence a renegotiation of fundamental disturbances in the self–other relation, they seek a path to independence. However, some people in analysis, violently abandon higher-level functioning in immediate transferential response to the analyst and demand care and reparation from the environment; their regression is very likely to be malignant.

A regression is malignant if the patient seeks self devolution in order to coerce an other – in this case the analyst – into unconditional care. The analyst is meant to be there on demand, for as long as needed, and in whatever way the patient determines. The condition is malignant because there is no unconscious intention of returning the self to independence. On the contrary, the analysis is regarded as the fulfilment of a promise made by the monsters of the environment to make their bad behaviour up to this patient by providing an object that would constitute class-action reparation.

Schizophrenic patients will often regress in violent ways, abandoning all self control, and perhaps insisting that the analyst look after them. Chronically depressed patients will also seek such interpersonal asylums in which they pressure the analyst to look after them. One can speak, then, of these situations as often – though by no means always – being malignant regressions, with the analysand using the analytical space as an end in itself and having no intention of returning the self to the world.

But the schizophrenic and the depressive (amongst others) usually give the analyst fair warning of his or her intention, and analysts have the opportunity to engage the patient's ideas over the course of some time. This is not so with the malignant hysteric, who often takes the analyst by surprise, and it is one of the reasons why in a clinic setting, for example, when analysts *think* one of the newcomers may be such a patient the intake team becomes unusually anxious.

Perhaps this is because so often the patient arrives in a state of obvious desperation. Perhaps it is because he often searches the faces of those who greet him with anguished and skilful gaze. Perhaps it is because the patient verbalises his or her plight with such evocative power and seems so precariously perched in reality. Certainly, it is distressing when he or she begs not to be rejected by the analyst, not to be abandoned by the world. Certainly, it is disarming when he or she says that he promises to do whatever the analyst requests. Certainly, it is unusual when he or she passionately confirms the analyst's observations.

Here is how one analyst described the first consultation with such a patient.

> I was on duty when she was referred up to my room and when she stood at the door I was immediately struck by the bizarre way she looked. She looked like someone who had come from a sixties outdoor wedding that had been rained out, so on the one hand she looked colourful and pretty in a sort of way, but also seemed like she had been drenched. Her lipstick was slightly askew, her mascara had run, there was a tear in her dress, her shoes were partly broken, and instead of a purse, she had a slightly worn but beautiful Liberty's bag. She immediately called me by my first name, complimented me on my office, sat in my chair, and without pausing told me she was in a terrible mess, said she assumed we had fifty minutes and would tell me everything as fast as she could. I found the account of her immediate life circumstances deeply moving and worrying. She was in a terrible crisis at work and in her love life. She searched my face in a way that is unforgettable and when I said something – I recall saying that I thought she hurried herself as if she believed she would never have the proper time to tell anyone about herself – she burst into tears of gratitude and said 'yes that's true, that's absolutely true' in a way that made me feel unrealistically bonded to her. As the session proceeded I was dominated by two completely different states of mind. On the one hand, I found her immensely appealing and deeply moving, and totally in need of help. On the other hand, she scared the hell out of me and I was wondering whatever was I going to do with her, and who could I find to 'take her on'.

This analyst, although young, was not clinically inexperienced. But he noted that with this patient there was a different type of transference in which he felt profoundly over-involved with the analysand, even though he feared her. He repeatedly emphasised her way of looking at him.

What he experienced was her *effect* upon him and the way the hysteric transforms the self into an event (see Chapter 9). The malignant hysteric believes that it is only through being 'effective' that the other will 'listen' and take the self into consideration. The other must be taken captive, must suffer the consequences of being in captivity and must believe that any future is in the hands of fate. To convey these views, the malignant hysteric will act in and act out in almost equal doses, as soon as analysis begins, coercing the analyst into being a paralysed witness to what seems an almost terrifying course of events, that not only draw the analyst into the situation, but suggest a dire fate.

In a sense, the malignant hysteric passes on to the other those parental projective identifications that have been communicated to the hysteric in the first place, from the mother, and also very possibly from the father. As discussed in Chapter 1, maternal projective identification is essential to the baby's psychic development. If this contact, however, is operating as a substitute for sensual engagement of the infant, such that maternal projective identification is the only form of touch, then the infant will be disposed to overvalue such inner effects. Further, as with the malignant hysteric, if the mother is the intermediary of her parent's evacuative projective identifications, then she too will violently project her inner objects into her child, who will be possessed by them. This is the aetiology of hysterical possession by foreign and invading spirits. Malignant hysterics feel displaced by a melange of others who have long since crowded out the self by their cacophonous, exacting nature. In hysterical psychosis one sees the self emptying itself of these objects, thing presentations operating under the thin veil of language.

The hysteric's surprise at what he or she contains, often a prelude to self dissociations, seems psychic testimony to this registration of parentally projected objects, long resident within the self. How do we name these internal objects, the ones constructed by the other inside the lexicon of the self's inner object world? For these are not introjects, but the other's projects. Elsewhere I have suggested that we name such internal objects *interjects*[1] to distinguish their psychic origin, status and future from the introject. An interject is that object projected into a self by the other which interrupts and momentarily disorients the self, which can proceed only insofar as it accepts the interjection. The dissociative state of the hysteric testifies to the act of self interruption. The seemingly affective surprise of the hysteric registers the shock over what is found inside.

Let us move on by considering a clinical example provided by an experienced therapist.

> When I first took on Sydney in psychotherapy, I knew this was not going to be easy, as he was volatile, intelligent, and 'innocent', and he said he felt at times 'possessed' by his 'demons'. In the second session he arrived an hour early and sobbed so loudly in the waiting room that the previous patient and I were made anxious by this and I did not know whether to go or to stay. But when I saw him, he was 'serenely calm', almost beatific, and he made no mention of his sobbing. Five minutes into the hour, however, and he turned over on the couch, looked intently at me, and then said that he wanted to feel his penis's impact on the couch; he wanted to feel himself 'grinding into analysis' and he

said, 'I promise I will not fail to discuss my sexuality. I know you need my experience in here, don't you!' and then he turned over on his back, said in a different tone of voice 'but I should behave myself' and went on to another subject.

I took up with him what he was doing, telling him that I thought he sought to substitute actions for words and to bring about in me an anxiety about what to expect from him. He replied that he was 'in analysis' and he did not care what effect he had on me as he only intended to talk to me about himself. If I was affected he was sorry but he could not let my feelings get in his way.

After the hour, which seemed both bizarre yet crafted, I was left wondering if indeed this was an hysteric and was I to be the object of hysterical disorder. I did not have to wait long. The next session he decided I needed to meet his best female friend, and he brought her to the hour, and was irritated that I would not see both of them together. Every so often he would attack me for being a stupidly cold 'shrink', but immediately – and bizarrely – apologise, all the while looking at me to see what I was making of this. I said as much. He said 'you do not believe me?', implying that I thought this was only an invention and then he fled from the hour. That night he left a message on my answering machine saying he did not think he could go on any longer with life and before hanging up banged the receiver about a few times. I was left worried and alarmed about his safety. He showed up for the next hour as if nothing had happened.

What this therapist then went on to describe was a series of such actings out which continuously disarmed him. He sought to talk matters through, only to find the patient was equally determined to prove that talking was the hope of fools, and would be displaced by actions that speak far louder than words. At a point when the patient seemed decompensated the therapist undertook involuntary hospitalisation, which was ineffective, as upon admission assessment the patient was calm and lucid, and discussed this 'incident' as the actions of an inexperienced and overly anxious therapist who 'should know better'. The hospital staff agreed with the patient.

In this first year of work there were to be many enactments as the patient 'infiltrated' the analyst's life – from finding out his wife's place of work and 'bumping into her', to finding out the children's school and giving them bouquets; from attending professional meetings where the therapist delivered a paper and where the patient rose from the audience to make a rebuttal, to writing passionate replies to critics of psychoanalysis, declaring that his analyst was living proof of the selfless and intelligent work of the psychoanalyst.

Not a week went by without the analyst feeling this patient's violation of his privacy and his own fear of what the patient might do. At the same time, he had dismissed what he considered very worrying diagnostic understandings. Although at times apparently psychotic, manic and psychopathic, the patient was not regarded as either borderline, schizophrenic, manic depressive or psychopathic, precisely because each of these diagnostic possibilities seemed momentary and, furthermore, stage-managed. The analyst felt that the patient was watching him endure each of these unfolding possibilities and, although he was very anxious at times, he also found this man unnervingly engaging and endearing. He had strong wishes to rescue the patient from himself.

Several months into treatment the clinician realised that the patient interpreted the analytic situation as a promise that could be exploited to a certain end: the analyst, and the 'promise' that is psychoanalysis, could be employed as a witness of a bizarre type of enacted testimonial, in which the self dangerously unravels its innards. In one period of ten days, the patient resigned from his job, stopped eating, and stood vigil outside the House of Commons in protest against a certain piece of legislation. Although he was hypomanic during this period, each action served momentarily to realise an inner presence – what he called important repressed parts of himself – as he acted them out. As a self-appointed medium of his own internal objects, he looked stricken and exhausted when he arrived for his analytic hours. He said he did not know how long he could survive and the analyst found that each time he made a comment his patient changed facial expression, posture and tone of voice. In the course of fifty minutes he manifested something like ten differing selves.

The analyst stood his ground, however, and told the patient that he seemed to think he could hold the analyst hostage to being a pure witness to mad scenes in which any attempt to speak would only create more madness. The analyst remained calm, undramatic and interpretive. He said that he knew the patient came from a family where the parents regularly enacted their mad scenes in the presence of the children and that he believed the patient was showing him this. When this brought up a new facial–bodily–vocal self he replied that the patient reckoned he could coerce his analyst into believing that he himself was no longer there, but was now inhabited by many others. He said he thought the patient was intoxicated by the idea that, like mother and father, he could enact whatever crossed his mind without consequence, and said that the patient now thought he had found a witness, helpless though he was, as a child upon whom to inflict each of these happenings.

No single case typifies the character disorder it is meant to represent. But clinicians who work with malignant hysteria will note certain features in this patient's presentation in common with those of other malignant hysterics and the problems raised in working with them.

As we have seen, these patients use the opportunity which analysis provides to receive their enactments but exploit this as an end in itself. They seek to drive the analyst into a helpless state wherein he or she is meant to witness a parade of characters and events which reconstitute in the analyst's countertransference the child's experience of overwhelming sexuality. Unlike the borderline patient, who seeks effectively to bond with the analyst in a fusion of turbulence, thus constituting the primary object, the malignant hysteric seeks to impose an inequality upon this dyad, in which a helpless and paralysed self is further enervated by the passing by of powerful visual scenes.

To an extent, the malignant hysteric displays a confusion between wakeful perceptions and dream-like representations, creating indigestible dream scenes which challenge the ability of any wakeful person to transform them into meaning. They are not meant to be so transformed, but instead to be terminal[2] objects that stick inside the self as unforgettable hauntings of past others and events.

In this respect we may see an insistence upon the imaginary order in defiance of the symbolic order, a militant presentation of scene upon scene upon scene, which visually overpowers anything like a verbal associative process. The malignant hysteric believes that the self is caught up in such an imaginary order, directed by an other equally possessed. The acute sense of the visual is important, as these patients seek visual impact as a thing in itself, and in this respect they merge the imaginary and the real, so that the witness watches not the movement of the imaginary as a field of illusionary representations of those who are absent, but as the scene-making order itself – the movement of a kind of god who displaces (or annihilates) any self aiming to imagine anything, as the presented scenes become equivalents to any reality. What the hysteric presents are not imagined scenes, then, but thing presentations of the self's early experience of the seen, which overpowered the senses and the psyche.

Think of it in terms of the mirror stage. Instead of experiencing an image of the self as a bound or complete speculation of the other, the hysteric gazing at the mirror is confronted with moving images or motion pictures. The maternal imaginary, overflowing with representations of its internal objects, acts them out upon the other, so that the mirror is now handed over to the child, who is meant to reflect the mother. Looking into the maternal mirror the child not only does not see a reflection of the self (instead, the mother's emptying of her internal world) but the child is used by the mother to see how she affects – i.e. is mirrored by – her child.

In analysis the malignant hysteric immediately dismantles the self, so that the clinician looks into a mirror – held by the patient – which releases into reality spectral images that should otherwise be held in the patient and talked into reality. Enacted in reality, the imaginary is transformed into the real, and the analyst is now living at the intersection of a violent collision between all of the orders, as both the imaginary and the symbolic are conflated by their change of function into materialisations of the real, moving through a self like a tornado ripping apart a landscape. The sheer force of this hysteric's presentations usurps its contents.

Transferentially, then, the malignant hysteric brings a psychotic-type reality to the analytical setting, overpowering the self with images and words functioning as the real. All along, however, this is an erotic reverie inherited from the mother's narrations and enactments. It is a bizarre means of sexually exploiting internal objects at the expense of actual others. As the internal is erotically articulated, the witness–other is paralysed with fear. This reverses the original conflict when the mother found the actual body of the infant, and especially the genitalia, too physically repulsive to transform imaginatively. Instead, the mother-become-malignant turns to an internal object that bears the name of her infant, and erotises the child. Not only does she erotise all of her internal objects, but the process of object formation itself is sexualised. In her relations to her child, to her other children, to her husband, she enacts scenes of erotic intensity that have a chilling effect upon the others.

This chilling effect occupies the analyst. And it is part of the analyst's task to interpret how the malignant hysteric deconstructs his or her person in order to intensify expressed internality in a defiant erotic exhibition of desire that refuses and annuls the other. It is part of the task to point out what it means that one's expression of desire should neutralise another's desire. It is part of the task to indicate what it means that the imaginary is only supposed to have impact and not be transformed into meaning. And it is part of the task to indicate through speech the power of the word to transform the image.

The hysteric has not experienced the mother's narrations and enactments as *from* the mother, but as *through* her. She is seen as a medium of powerful and terrifying forces moving through her body. These forces are not only indistinguishable from the impact of the instincts, they constitute the representation of the instinct. The power of instinctual states has seemingly occupied the mother from within and driven through her body with *its* mental representations – rather like Freud's theory of the instinct that chooses its object solely on the grounds of expediency. For Freud, the instinct chooses its object in a totally arbitrary way and the mother of the malignant hysteric stands as outraged witness to this very process, showing the self's experience of being driven by instinct.

Malignant hysterics empty themselves into the analytical holding space as a violent force that transfers their psychic status as mediums of the sexual instinct. Even seasoned analysts treating malignant hysterics experience an unprecedented level of fear, unknown with borderline or schizophrenic patients. These psychic 'cousins' may be more impaired, but the hysteric is remarkably skilled at portraying the self and its inner dilemma. They may present as borderline or schizophrenic (or as having other character disorders), but the hysteric's particular skill is to get inside the other and enact that other's character – a skill which is unnerving when it operates malignantly, portraying the dismantling of erotic life, the violent movements of displacement as a function of the drive, in which the scenes conveyed to the analyst present the sexual as dementing.

A patient, and her psychotherapist.

Judy was a 27-year-old woman when she entered hospital for the third time. She was diagnosed as borderline because she was, amongst other things, impulsive, given to manic flights of affect, easily enraged, infantile and inclined to throw off boundaries.

When she entered a room, even if calm, she always suggested that she could transform herself from what looked like an attractive and ordinary human being into a possessed figure, deeply demented and driven by forces she never even saw, much less contained. So when she entered the patients' lounge, for example, she would walk up to a vase, lift it in a way that suggested she might then throw it against the wall, but then calmly replace it. Or she might walk into a room with ten chairs and several couches, and sit on the same couch occupied by one of only four people sitting in the room, in a way that suggested she was up to something. Or whilst others were watching a particular television programme, she might walk up to the table where the television guide lay and pick it up, glancing at it intently, indicating that she might abruptly change the channel. Such ideas would occur to the group because on previous occasions she had picked up an object and thrown it against the wall, she had sat next to a patient and then punched him in the groin, and she had abruptly changed the television channel. The group began to suffer its reminiscences.

Part of what was so disconcerting was that her 'attacks', as they were called, were so sudden. The group was paralysed and even the staff were thrown into momentary enervation. Furthermore, she could – and occasionally did – suddenly desist, right in the midst of a tempest. For example, one day she threw strawberries across the room, yelled insulting remarks about the cook, and shoved another patient against the wall, but suddenly stopped. The room about her was a hive of flight and recuperatory activity, frozen by her cessation. She calmly walked away from the scene and entered the lounge. An amiable member of staff gave her a few minutes and then walked into the room and sat with her in silence before venturing to speak. He told the staff later that he was frightened to speak for fear it might 'set her off'.

But the anxiety of speaking *to* such a person is a common anxiety in the clinician, who also fears that speech might evoke a sudden outburst of scene-making. And if the ordinary hysteric transforms himself or herself momentarily into an event, watched by an observant ego to its own pleasure, the malignant hysteric's same self-observation is much more bizarre. Although the malignant hysteric witnesses himself or herself as an unfolding scene, he or she is split off into that infant or child self for whom the mirror reveals not the image of one's self, but its own hidden internal objects, passed off as one's self. The malignant hysteric who witnesses the self as evolving chaos observes something more like the pure force of the instinct choosing objects in spite of the self and the other, shoving the relational aside in the wake of the instinct's path.

If we take an ordinary instinct such as thirst, for example, let us imagine that whilst the self is out gardening on a hot day the instinct forces the mind to think, 'I am thirsty.' Perhaps the self will say, 'I would like a drink of water.' The object of the instinct and the object that will please the self are compatible. Imagine a different instinct in a more complex setting. The self has a full bladder, giving rise to the instinct to urinate, and the self thinks, 'I need to urinate.' The aim of the instinct is to urinate and the object of the instinct would be that idea through which such a pressure could be imaginatively extinguished. So the object might be, 'I need to go to the toilet.' Once again, the object of the instinct and the self's actual fulfilment of it are compatible: a toilet can be found. But what if the same instinct – let's say in a man – gives rise to the following thought: 'I need to pee on my foot.' Why would the instinct choose *that* object? Because each instinct will have had its own peculiar history 'in' each self and in the example I have selected, the self has changed the customary object for a different one. What if the same instinct is represented through the following: 'I need a woman to pee on my foot, whilst I am being called an ungrateful asshole'? What one sees here is that the instinct and its history constitute the self's sexuality, which over time records and becomes the subject's desire.

For reasons described in previous chapters, the hysteric regards the sources of sexuality – especially the genitalia – as disturbing, and there is a feeling that it is disruptive and vile. The mother of a malignant hysteric experiences sexual mental contents as violently determined by the drive, with which she refuses to associate. Her dissociation is intense and effective, as she transfers them from inside herself to her external world through forms of narrative and performance, although, as mentioned before, the specific mental contents will have been displaced, so that she is transferring seemingly non-sexual states of mind into the outside world by narrative–performative expulsion. When the hysteric observes himself or herself or observes the analyst relating to him or her, he or she is watching the effect of drives upon the mind, indicating why and how they can wreak havoc with human lives.

When Judy walked into a room she created an illusion that she would be unable to contain herself should she ever be occupied by the drives. She also created the illusion that much of the time she was drive free, suspended for a time, or in a more petrified state of mind. She would, for example, sit in one position for hours, looking very calm and serene. Passers-by would be as unnerved by this as they would be by her more tempestuous states. But, unlike the schizophrenic's catatonic serenity, derived from a killing-off of mental functions that might process the drives, the hysteric's statuesque calm is only the curtain lowered in an interval that announces the certainty of another outbreak of the self's inner life, one that will leave the world caught up in a sexual turmoil. As such, the serenity and its opposite are linked, just as Lot's now petrified wife is linked to the forbidden sexual scene upon which she gazed.

In the preceding chapter, following Freud's theory of infantile sexuality, we suggested that hysterical regression involves a return to polymorphous sexuality, in which the component instincts seem cut loose from the integrations imposed by genital organisation. In subtle or gross ways, for example, Judy would release these instincts to fellow patients and clinicians. She would pee on the floor, often giggling uncontrollably, and fart and celebrate the odour – gross offences to the group. At the dinner table there were times when she would eat by smacking her lips, holding the food in her mouth for long periods before swallowing, sucking solids off a spoon, or putting her hands in the dish to play with mashed potatoes or salad. Perhaps we could term this the mid-grotesque. In a more subtle vein, however, she would gaze at a man or woman with an equal quality of ravenous licentiousness, or she would call to someone with sonic seductiveness, releasing her voice into the group as an auditory instinct seeking some hapless sex object. In one day alone she could be all of these things, a moving theatre of the infantile, celebrating the polymorphous.

The malignant hysteric seeks a formal regression, a regression in the basic form of the self, from higher-level functioning to something else – which I hesitate to term lower-level functioning. The formal change is to absent the self as the recipient of the instincts and move it slightly to the side – from associate to dissociate – as the drive now arrives pure and simple in its disturbing choice of object. Judy once reached over very calmly and put her hand on another patient's breast as if she were in a trance and her hand was being guided by a force over which she not only had no control but no knowledge. When she masturbated in public it was as if another's hand was performing the action.

Such patients try to convince the analyst that whatever they release in this presence is not of their making even if it derives from them. They implore the analyst not to reject them, for 'they know not what they do'. In North America such personalities are finding paradoxical refuge in the category of multiple personality, where clinicians, when agreeing to talk to different alters, implicitly accept the fate of a self which is absent at the moment of mental release. In the spiralling regressions typical of such patients, as they release inner states which effectively destroy conventional self functioning and intimate relations with the other, they indicate that original experience of being at the mercy of one's own drives.

One of the best illustrations of malignant hysteria in the literature is in Harold Stewart's essay 'Problems of management and communication' (1992). Referred by a colleague from hospital, Stewart's young patient 'looked rather wild and scruffy, wore torn jeans' (p. 84) and complained of depressions that had begun some ten years ago after her first sexual experience. We may speculate that the depression registered the unconscious catastrophe posed by sexuality itself, which, as I have argued, results in the destruction of the hysteric's relation to the mother.

Stewart's patient felt unloved, was having an affair with a married man in which she was sexually subservient yet frigid, possessed little sense of self, wanted to be a man, and 'was a compulsive clitoral masturbator' (p. 84). She held her father in contempt and feared her mother, who used to burst into wild physical acts of violence during her childhood and then blame the children for causing these outbursts. She did have a kind maternal grandmother to whom she was close, although the grandmother saw ghosts and had a tenuous hold on reality.

In the beginning of the analysis the patient would be good for several sessions and then suddenly burst into provocative and scathing verbal attacks, for which she apologised. Stewart understood these outbursts as cautious testings of his capability. She then became more infantile and acted out physically in sessions by trying to grab his penis. For a very long period of time she was preoccupied with the analyst's genitals and when trying to grab them would be met by his physical holding of her.

Stewart does not write this paper to discuss hysteria per se, but focuses on management issues. He notes that there are certain patients – and this patient is one of them – for whom verbal intervention would not have sufficed and for whom a physical form of holding had to take place. He mentions but does not elaborate his countertransference, but it is not difficult to imagine from his account of the patient the imaginative turmoil that he had to undergo during her analysis. We may consider his physical intervention as an important symbolic action as he brought the body of the other to the patient for the binding of sexual states of mind. In the course of her regression in treatment the patient developed delusional and hallucinatory ideas of her sexuality, which we may understand as the inevitable effect of sexuality upon a mind desperate to avoid it.

The analyst must, then, bind sexuality – which Stewart does by physically restraining his patient – so that it might find another route of expression, which in this case it does as the patient turns to drawing and painting as a medium of self expression. It also seems to release her to intensified hallucinatory states, for example, when she talked about 'a persistent vision of her genitals rotting away'. Stewart tells us: 'On putting her hand there' – referring to her genitals – 'she felt a large hole where they had rotted away and was terrified' (p. 92). She realised this was a negative hallucination and then touched herself to rediscover their existence. We may interpret this hallucination as the outcome of her attack on her genitals, which, as an hysteric, she understands as the root cause of her loss of a loving world.

Later in the analysis, during dark winter evenings, the patient entered a type of reverie and wanted only one light on in the consulting room, demanding absolute quiet. If Stewart stirred she accused him of masturbating. She had fantasies of sucking his penis, his breast, her thumb and of masturbating. She actually did masturbate and then was shocked at what she had done. There was confusion over who was manipulating whose genitals. We may see, however, that the patient had regressed to a place where she could express her confusion over who controls the scenery of the erotic, given her conviction that erotic life derives exclusively from any self's auto-erotic interests. In the presence of the other she is unclear whether her sexual self-stimulations or the other's sexual self-stimulations will determine the course of sexuality between the two.

This patient recovered from her analysis, went on to marry and find a profession, and the case report ends with her expressed wish to have children. Stewart takes up the controversy surrounding some of his techniques – especially physical restraint – but does not discuss what is probably obvious to any reader, namely, that success with this type of patient takes a great deal of clinical acumen. For every one of these patients who meets with a successful outcome from an analysis, there are unfortunately too many who do not profit from the experience, probably due to the analyst's lack of experience of work in this area. But, sadly enough, the malignant hysteric's unconscious need to sabotage the work of insight may also contribute to these failures. For 'looking into' is understood as the preferred option to 'acting out', which is unconsciously interpreted as a refusal of the patient's exhibition of the self, a 'showing' that is the self-as-genital, intended to captivate, control and subdue the other, who will accept that such mind-boggling theatricals are beyond control.

Another patient.

Roger was a smart university graduate who refused professional education and instead worked in a bookstore much of his life. A voracious reader, he fancied himself something of an expert in many differing fields. He was in a long-standing relation with Fred and they were very supportive of one another and well liked by their friends. Every so often, however, Fred would have to hospitalise Roger because of the latter's sudden toxic states of anxiety, which gave rise to manic and delusional states of mind. These would be announced by a sudden intensification of Roger's otherwise – at least so far as Fred was concerned – charming habit of believing he could 'enter' into a problem (or a person, or a couple, or a political issue, etc.) with special powers of intuition from which he could then deliver an oracle that would predict how things would be. He had studied astrology for a long time, could read anyone's chart, and had interests in paranormal phenomena and the like.

Fred had a hard time describing the quality of Roger's more intense imaginings, as they were somehow 'sexual' but he found it hard to say exactly in what way. Roger would go into a kind of trance, which he often did, but on these occasions he seemed transported by his very invocation of the medium. He became very dominating and demanding, and would caress his body and insist that his physical presence was vibrating with the effects of communicated truth. Fred said that it was like watching a porno film gone bad, or a porno plot that had left the director and was now walking loose in the world at large as a performance in itself. Roger seemed to have no idea of how he was coming across or of how out of hand things had become.

The casualty officer of the hospital, who had treated Roger on an intensive basis before, found him almost always in the same state: he was usually drenched in perspiration, wearing inappropriately revealing clothes, yet apparently oblivious to his self-presentation. He was rather offensively rude and grandiose, and talked in a loud and contemptuous voice and, as he was quite bright, his criticisms of staff and the hospital were often irritatingly accurate. He seemed to be in some sort of trance and appeared caught up in an erotic delusion in which he believed he was the centre of the universe – a kind of sexual centre – from which he could divine the future and pre-ordain the most important meetings to come. For example, he would now and then visit other patients in the waiting-room, touching them on the head or shoulders like a kind of sexual Pope giving benediction. He procured a drink from the dispenser and flourished his cup of water as though it were filled with elixir.

Although there are obvious manic symptoms to Roger's breakdown, he responded every time to heavy sedation and spent only two days at most in hospital. Once discharged, he was mildly embarrassed and yet charming and all was forgiven until his next episode. In fact, these episodes always followed his discovery of an important new author, or an interesting new field that he did not know about, and an intense period of immersive reading when he felt joined to the new object. This new discovery was sexualised, and he would then begin to act out in sexual ways that were otherwise atypical of him, alarming Fred, whom he treated with disdain.

When Roger entered intensive psychotherapy he broke down in the transference through deep intoxication with the analyst, whom Roger assumed he knew better than the analyst knew himself. He invented all kinds of words and concepts to explain the analyst to himself. He spoke in a special voice, which was a curious mixture of the intimate talk between lovers and aggressive coerciveness, oscillating between being affectionate and being threatening. In the course of his treatment it became clear that he regressed to an hysterical core in which he imagined himself the auto-erotic centre of the universe, always set off by his attempt to form a relation to a new-found object, which he then interpreted as having its 'vibration' – i.e. erotic core – which he could only fathom by merging with the object in what amounted to two self-stimulating orders in one. The aim of his communications to the other from that point on – Fred or the analyst – was to show that he did not need the other, indeed, that the other should take its own auto-erotic stimuli from Roger's pronouncements and then join him as a fellow self-stimulator in his orbit.

Roger experienced analytical interpretation as insulting. That he should develop insight into himself, rather than procure a licence for the export of his ideas, seemed to him ludicrous. Although his analyst was highly experienced, Roger was determined to set up a 'counter-analysis' in which each and every interpretation was to be transformed, if not into its opposite, then into an 'alternative', and sessions were at best like strange sporting events, with Roger matching the analyst's comments with his own views. In time the analyst was faced with a difficult decision. It became clear that whenever Roger was at risk of understanding something about himself, inevitably bringing him toward depressive anxieties, he would engage in violent self dismantlings, tearing himself into mental pieces. He would drink and take drugs, forgo sleep, and go on social binges that resulted in both physical and psychic emaciations that drove desperate forms of thought, always verging on the hallucinatory. The analyst knew that such dissolutions of the self were aimed at eradicating any reliable form of consciousness in order to rid the self of emergent insight. The analyst interpreted this, often commenting on how Roger took to self-destruction to ensure that he would always be an event beyond the influence of anyone other than himself. He aimed, so the analyst maintained, to keep the other in a state of enervated bewilderment, so that he could register his existence through the toxic effects on the other. The fact remained, however, that interpretation in itself did not mitigate this aspect of Roger's mental state, and as time went on it became very clear that the patient was hell-bent on further self dissolution.

When Roger talked frankly about suicide, partly to coerce the analyst, partly to terrify Fred, the analyst nonetheless took the threat as a serious possibility and arranged for a transfer to hospital, where Roger was placed for an extended period of time. The analysis did continue afterwards, but Roger was also in the care of a psychiatrist, who determined that he should be on maintenance medication for the remainder of his life, with the mixed result that the patient 'stabilised' but was in a somewhat permanent state of chemo-mediation, rather as if a perversion had been fashioned to foreclose the possibility of a neurosis. The analyst was distressed by this state of affairs, but the patient had pushed him – he told himself – to the limits of his capability and there was nothing that could be done to affect the situation.

Looking from the previous chapter to this – from the theatre of the hysteric to the malignant hysteric – we see a spectrum that we may locate in the self's experience of 'family life'. As we know, a self enters the family first through the maternal order, with the paternal order functioning as the third element: one which precedes the self's birth and waits for the child to emerge into language and naming. But 'family' is a fourth object, which includes the three existing orders, and is a different composition.

A family is a group to which the members belong and although bearing the father's name – i.e. 'the Smith family' – it is a small world. In the countless negotiations among members a family evokes its myths, legends, facts, history, aesthetics, visions and laws. Any child development is a self's movement into this world, internalising its constituent elements carried as an inner object to function in the name of the family. The self may reject its constituents, but it cannot erase its registration, so we shall carry with us our family's elements, which together become a composition.

Although family therapy exists as the first treatment programme for this object – and has produced very interesting texts – arguably we still have to think to ourselves what a family is. Certainly, this fourth object proves a puzzle to the hysteric. Driven to identify and represent the other's desire, destined therefore to oscillate between representing the inner worlds of mother and father, what does the hysteric do with the fourth object? By an act of discriminating internalisation, the elements of this world become cathected as sub-erotic phenomena, available for sexual reverie and later for erotic transmission. The hysteric takes the laws of the family as a set of interdictions that form an erotic matrix, an inner set carried by each hysteric into other families and later into the self's family, in order to employ it (or to impose it) as the desired set through which all other sets are filtered.

The hysteric, then, does not simply identify with and represent the inner worlds of the parents; he or she also expresses at certain moments the elements of his or her family, either acting out a family fact (such as a move or death), or engaging a family of others with the self's own fourth object as erotic object.

A patient.

Luciana was courted by Carlos and introduced to his family. They were both Catholics, from the same medium-sized town, and of the same social class. At first she seemed content with being a new member of Carlos's family, but not long after their wedding serious problems emerged. Luciana was very insistent that Carlos follow certain rules in the house, such as washing up the salad plates before sitting down for the next course, or hanging the bath mat on the side of the bath and not on a hanger. Each room of the house had certain laws. Luciana also had very particular tastes, in painting, decoration, music, clothing and literature.

Carlos had found this difference to be one of Luciana's attractions – she was so wonderfully unique. But Luciana rather violently removed Carlos's aesthetic objects from the house or complained about his tastes so vehemently that he put them away. For example, first thing in the morning Carlos loved to pick up the newspaper with his coffee and absorb himself in the sports page, but in Luciana's family the day began with a collective discussion of what to do that day, followed by preparations for departure. Newspaper reading was done at the end of the day, after the dishes were washed and the house tidied.

Carlos wondered why Luciana could not tolerate at least 'some' of his ways. When interviewed by a marital therapist, the therapist wondered if Luciana was an obsessive or a narcissist. What could not be seen at first was Luciana's 'remembering' of her fourth object as a structure, a recalling of a set which brought its sub-erotic elements into an erotic object that sustained her reveries during the day. She had also insisted that each day she recall an aspect of her family's history, or tell one of her family's stories, often musing on her family's visions of reality and the future.

Everyone but the psychotic personality internalises the fourth object, but only the hysteric cathects it as an erotic object to serve as a matrix for subsequent defensive experiencing. What we call family life is the movement in space and time of this fourth object, of which the self is a member. For the hysteric, being a family member is an erotic expression, as the self – already dispersed in acts of representative identification – is further disseminated by the logic of the constellation of which the hysteric is a working member.

Most ordinary people rarely give this any thought and do not activate the sub-erotic elements of the fourth object. It is part of the self's ego – a part of its way of processing lived experience – along with other internal objects that constitute self experiencing. But the hysteric feels driven to express this object when in a fourth space or thinking about a fourth space. Some of the thoughtless perambulations of the hysteric in the household are forms of remembering the fourth object, constituting the matrix of an erotic reverie which always feeds the secret agony or the self's pining for its past.

Helena, another patient, walked through her house, dusting and arranging its contents in a daydreaming motion. These contents – her family's objects – were erotic members of the sense of the family, and as she walked into the different rooms – living-room, library, kitchen, laundry, children's room, bedroom – she entered space that suggested many things. She followed differing paths, according to her sense of the moment, quite content to commune in her family space. However, her walkings were always in the circles of her home, tracing and retracing footsteps.

The hysteric cannot accept his or her destiny as the unconscious articulation of the self's idiom through the use of objects, but instead has erotised his or her fate as the order into which one was born and through which one was predestined. Even as he or she repeatedly institutes the auto-erotism of fate as opposed to the allo-erotism of destiny (as fate repeats the self in easily recognised patterns and destiny opens the self to its infinite diversities), the hysteric may betray a form of rage against this narrowing of the self and its relations. Thus, there is a curious rage blending into the hysteric's auto-erotics, infiltrating representations of the fourth object with a certain violence. It is not simply an attempted cancellation of the other's fourth object – which is often accomplished – but a bitterly unconscious eradication of the self's diverse potential, a form of suicide by family identification. It is as if the self says: 'I am deferred as a member of this royal court, from which I derive my power and position. My own personal desires – whatever they might be – are to be set aside in the interests of participation in the royal family.'

To some extent this is each person's struggle. How am I defined by my family? If I have belonged to it, what was this act of belonging? And, if I differ from it, what are the terms of the difference? Perhaps for many, the self's idiom – always a singular intelligence of form – has long since differed from all others, and although it uses common objects (including the family) it does so idiosyncratically, creating its colloquial dialect in being. The hysteric, however, fights against this differing because the articulating destiny of idiom seems to separate the self from its family of origin. Part of the technique of resistance is the continuous theatre of remembrance as the hysteric enacts, again and again, parts of the family within a mentality that expresses the family matrix.

The analyst is to be found in the fourth object, a figure inside a mad family, whose intersecting internal worlds find a collecting logic of sorts in the family as group. He is inside an object that is the locality of a culture. He or she is a single thinker questioning an other who is only a medium for a group. Without knowing it, perhaps, the analyst is actually a group psychoanalyst when working with the malignant hysteric. By captivating the analyst in the topsy-turvy world of enactments, the hysteric teaches the analyst what it is like to find one's true self masticated by group madness. Like the hysteric, the analyst looks to this other to see himself or herself. Often, it is not a matter of choice, as the group of the patient's transferential object representations is so bizarre that the analyst is at a loss to find out which part of him or her is being addressed by the patient. The hysteric will subvert the analyst's ordinary relation to reconstructions. In work with other patients the analyst listens to the patient's history – and recalls the history of the analytical sessions as well – in order to find unconscious nourishment from these sources. Out of the past one finds the present and its future. The malignant hysteric presents a bewildering fourth object, which necessitates history-taking, of the patient's family and, more importantly, an intense recollection of analytical sessions. In trying to answer the questions 'What does this mean?', and 'Where are these communications coming from?' the analyst sinks into the past, from which it is not intended that he or she will return. Like the hysteric before the fourth object, the analyst is meant to drown in the sorrows of the past, to be swept up in the agonies of the ancestors. It is intended that the analyst will never find his or her place in the present, and the future is meant to evaporate as an imaginative possibility. More than a few psychoanalysts, when they reach this point in the analysis, end treatment or send the patient on to a colleague for another analysis.

As with the Siren seducing Odysseus, hysterical narrative–performance is meant to entrap any self that would assume its intended journey. Knowing that psychoanalysis is his or her co-invention, the hysteric assumes possession of the psychoanalyst, and demands that the analyst sacrifice his or her own personal ambitions to the violent charms of the other. The analyst is meant to be spellbound and shipwrecked. He or she is meant to give up the profession. As we shall see in the next chapter, the hysteric becomes addicted to the transference, and, as we shall discuss in Chapter 13, he or she insists that the analysis become sexualised and the analyst become its victim.

When hysterics become psychotic they abandon themselves to the many characters whom they have contained. With unnerving skill, they hallucinate or act out in a fugue-hallucinatory manner a small colony of others. The so-called multiple personality is a kind of charade of hysterical psychosis, giving each character a seemingly complete and full identity. The hysteric who presents as a multiple seeks a doctor who desires a patient's illness as the form of his own phallic empowerment. The hysteric will be the maternal phallus, acting out the psychoanalyst's desire.

Hysterical psychosis is a particular form of decompensation in which the self stands to one side, as it were, and projects scenes through the actions of the self's body. An eerie feature of this psychosis is that the patient witnesses himself or herself in his or her madness, creating the illusion that the psychosis is directed by a psychotic voyeur, who gains satisfaction at the sight of the self impacting the other – a primal scene created by the imaginary which impresses itself upon the real. The psychosis intends to reverse the process of internalisation. Internal contents are meant to project themselves into the environment, transforming the imagery of the real into reflections of the hysteric's inner life. The violence of this intended projection is unconscious revenge against its opposite: the self's sufferings from its own internalisations. Indeed, the world is now meant to suffer its own agony of reception, as the other is intended to be overwhelmed by the self's internal world.

Hysterical psychosis presents undigested images, visual scenes that defy meaning, because any self is meant to forget them in self-protection. Clinicians working with the psychotic actions of the hysteric do indeed find them very hard to think about, precisely because the hysteric has presented himself or herself in a grotesquely vivid manner. This is a kind of sexual psychosis, as the patient wraps these scenes in sexual lining, all too often driving the analyst into further bewilderment by an erotism gone awry. Scene follows scene, and character follows character in bits and pieces across the hysteric's stage. No schizophrenic shows such directorial skill; no schizophrenic could ever portray all the psychoses in one single performance; no borderline patient's psychotic regression is accompanied by a split-off part of the patient sitting in as a revelling audience; and yet, even in the midst of the most bizarrely psychotic states, the hysteric watches the psychosis-as-primal-scene. For this is a psychosis that represents sexuality. Sexuality that drives the self mad. An intercourse that blinds any witness, that forces the other to avert its gaze.

In this respect hysterics-in-psychosis pose the one scene they cannot bear. They can look upon the depressed mother. They can watch the enraged father. They can bear loss of the other, whether it leaves them off at school, or whether it dies. Yet none of them wants to bear witness to parental intercourse. The idea – much less the sight – is unthinkable. In a psychotic way? No. This is not an attack on linking as such, that is to say, an attack on the very perceptual apparatus. Rather, this is an assault on a very particular idea, or more properly, a sight-idea. This is what Iago calls the 'beast with two backs', the sight of a monster, that drives the child into a sense of horror over what he or she sees. Hysterical psychosis always portrays violating intercourse. Between the warring characters in hysterical theatre one finds representation of violent intercourse between male and female characteristics.

Set against this opera of grotesqueries is the other side of hysterical psychosis, what Donnet and Green (1973) call a 'blank psychosis', although I use the term here in a somewhat different way. For in the midst of seemingly uncontrollable madness, the hysteric can suddenly cease all representations and return to remarkable lucidity – back to normality, then, or into blank psychosis: into an elected mutism, body often rigid, self immobile, gaze fixed, and sonic attention closed off. In this opposition one sees, as discussed in earlier chapters, the other hysteric route, that driven by the death drive. In this ascetic hysteria one finds the self returned to its deep freeze, the precocity of florid psychotic representations completely silenced. The juxtaposition of these two self states – florid psychosis/ blank psychosis – expresses a different type of intercourse, one between the cold anti-sexual self and the sexually possessed. Between the violence of the nun and the violence of the prostitute, the hysteric lives – a directorial presence that transcends its represented extremes.

More than a few psychoanalysts have hoped to speak to the hysteric off stage. More than a few psychoanalysts have felt privileged with what they take to be an audience with the director. But betrayal is the name of the game. The hysteric takes the other into trust in order to break it before the eyes of the other. How many clinicians, having worked diligently and apparently with success, have brought the psychotic hysteric to a point of apparent psychic change, only to have this belief shattered, often in a very public way? How many clinicians have returned from holiday to find that the patient who has made so much apparent progress has in fact attempted suicide?

Trust built on reciprocity often feels like an insult to the hysteric. It seems like a lie. Such trust is the work of suckers, people lulled into infant-like soporifics. Such trusts should be busted up. They should be violated by the sights and sounds of another coupling, one that is all wrapped up in itself, one that refuses the meaningful participation of any other. Becoming this beast with two backs, the hysteric-in-psychosis breaks up the therapeutic alliance by means of the auto-erotic primal scene, a vision of a self fucking itself up, enclosed in a mad embrace that defies any other to intervene.

We are unlikely to know how many of the diagnosed schizophrenics, manic depressives and borderlines in mental hospitals are in fact malignant hysterics. The very fact that psychoanalysis, infatuated with psychiatric categories after the

Second World War, desired 'primitive mental states' in the form of the borderline, has meant that hysterics would always satisfy this desire, especially as it promised progeny out of the psychotic primal scene. Each analyst engaged in these new intercourses felt he or she was at a new frontier, espying a new psychic entity, ready for its writing and its naming. The fact that psychoanalysis in hospitals gradually expunged hysteria from its lists meant that it had to reappear in other forms.

We shall continue our discussion of psychosis and hysteria in the last chapter of the book. But now we turn to a more common form: the hysteric who inhabits psychoanalysis as an alternative to living.

Notes

1   For further discussion of this concept see my *The Mystery of Things* (Bollas, 1999).
2   For further discussion of this concept, see my *Cracking Up* (Bollas, 1995).

Chapter 12

Transference addicts

Looking back at the patients in *Studies on Hysteria* one finds that as soon as they produce a new set of symptoms, which Freud then analyses, they create another set of symptoms, which in turn demand a new set of interpretations. Frau Emmy, for example, would present him with disturbing pictures; he would seek their origin through diligent questioning, and then use hypnosis to 'wipe out all these memories' (Breuer and Freud, 1893: 59). In subsequent writings Freud would look back on these first studies and regard himself as rather naive, proposing to the reader that subsequent understandings removed the obstacles repeatedly established by the patient. He certainly did learn a great deal more, but he captured something in these early writings that is accurate and still very puzzling.

Psychoanalysts are as averse as anyone else to writing up their failures, but if they felt free to do this then the literature would be amply populated by a certain type of hysteric who defeats the analytical process and brings about an unsuccessful end to analysis. To get to the heart of the matter, I am obviously leaving aside those failures that are the analyst's primary responsibility.

I shall begin with a brief clinical history.

Anastasia had two psychotherapies and three analyses lasting from her late twenties until her late sixties. There were breaks in the treatment, especially after one analysis in which the analyst had taken the view that the patient needed no further treatment. But other than this, she was always on the couch.

For the first decades she was seen as a very frustrating person who complained of a virtual cessation of meaning in her family and career, and was remarkably unwilling to get down to analytical work. One analyst resigned from treatment on the grounds that she was unanalysable, but this was early on in her analytical career. Another, who analysed her for ten years, found her initially very tight-lipped and uncooperative, except when complaining. Yet she had a rich dream life, which she reported in great detail, rather like gifts to some higher authority that would eventually translate them into great meaning. This analyst understood the extent of the patient's conscious revenge against him as she consistently refused to tell him what in fact was crossing her mind in his presence. Had she done so she would have been compelled to indicate that she was romantically preoccupied with him much of the time but otherwise deeply angry with him because she envied the people in his life. This included other patients, of course, but also members of his family and colleagues in his profession, and, although she was often in touch with her tender and passionate feelings for him, the sight of him was sufficient to arouse in her a deep fury and an intention to punish him by ruining his work as an analyst, and thus the analysis as well.

She had alluded to this on several occasions, however, so over time the analyst worked diligently in this area and some progress was made. It became clear that she intended the analysis to continue throughout her lifetime, ostensibly because of certain psychological ailments – which she articulated – but which unconsciously were directed toward the triumph of her exclusive relation to the analyst. She would be with him longer than anyone, longer than his wife and any other intimates. She was not going to give up her space to any other. There was to be no arrival of a sibling to displace her. She would remain and her illness was her claim on the territory.

It is at this point that we should discuss what is meant by the term 'entrenched hysteric'.

As we have discussed in the preceding chapters, the hysteric erotises absence. Absence of maternal touch is paradoxically erotised as the child senses that maternal abstention is derived from anxiety over temptations. The hysteric becomes furtive, operating through voice, gaze and ellipsis. What he or she eventually has is the symptom, and as with Freud's Emmy, Anastasia had herself as an object presented to the analytical other as the task of cure, as if saying: 'Here I am before your very eyes and within earshot. I place my inner life before you. I have no hope for myself, but you claim expertise: cure me.'

Each day that Freud analysed Emmy she conjured new symptoms to meet him the following day. Each of her therapists and analysts were given new sets of problems to solve. Certainly equal to the vivid presentations of Charcot's individuals in distress, Anastasia would break down in front of colleagues or friends, who became passionate advocates of her continued treatments.

With each new therapeutic undertaking Anastasia was a newborn, forming in her mind – and perhaps with her clinician's co-operation – a story about her previous analysis, inevitably highlighting its shortcomings, implicitly assigning to the new analyst the function of the better mother and father. By changing analysts throughout her lifetime she managed successfully to evade both conscious and unconscious engagement with the limits of existence and sustained a delusion that she was always a young girl, her life as an adult a long time ahead of her in the future. Anastasia's presenting of herself as incomplete was an invitation to the other's phallic entry, to fill her with more and more analytical knowledge, as semi-stuporous erotic supplicant to the virility of her analyst.

The entrenched hysteric's suffering is his or her passion. It is an expression of the patient's erotic life: to give up the symptom is equivalent to abandoning any erotic claim upon the object. It is a condensation of several factors. The patient remains untreatable, so in a certain way is always beyond the therapeutic arms of the clinician. This is the patient's presentation of absence, inherited from the mother and extended by the child. This absence is intended to affect the analyst, who is meant to share in the suffering of the occasion, which indeed he or she does. This presents the joining of two auto-sufferers, sharing a secret passion. The wish that it might be different, that life might emerge to displace this unending pain, is only to be held in joint separate states of mind, as the self and its other are meant to be at odds with one another. Separate yet equal.

The child's agony over being excluded by the mother is also incorporated in this passion and manifests itself in the form of the patient's presentation of new symptoms each time old ones have been worked through.

The suffering becomes an extension of the self: the psychic equivalent of the growth of a limb that can grasp and hold on to the other. Analytical interpretation that resolves any immediate complaint or symptomatic report is unconsciously experienced as a castration of this limb. Following a session in which the patient is almost forced to accept understanding – and it is very common that this patient, in the presence of the analyst, does indeed experience the sense of being understood – the patient works to undo the understanding, as this will allow the limb to remain extended.

These patients, then, often remain in treatment for the better part of a lifetime. Anastasia's use of analysis is unfortunately not uncommon, although commoner still are the patients who are in lifetime's treatment with people of differing therapeutic persuasions.

One woman, for example, was diagnosed as having an eating disorder in her late teens, whilst at university, and was in treatment with an expert in this field until her late twenties. Then she had a deep conviction that she must have been sexually molested when she was a child, and was referred to a specialist in this field with whom she worked until she was in her mid-thirties. At this time she developed alternative personalities and was referred to someone whose speciality was in the area of multiple personality disorder. She remained in treatment with him for nearly six years. All of these experts were in the same city. They knew of each other and referred patients to one another. They had access to clinics both in the city and in other states. The patient spent recuperation periods at centres for the treatment of eating disorders, sexual abuse and multiple personality disorder in other regions of the country, treated by colleagues of the experts looking after her. When she finally entered psychoanalytical psychotherapy it was obvious that this very intelligent woman had a deep investment in her illness and in promoting herself as ill.

We can understand this promotion if we see – as I think Freud did – that psycho-neurotic illness is an expression of the self's erotic life. To the casual observer (or even to an expert in one of mental health's sub-specialities), the idea that the patient's suffering is a form of desire will certainly seem odd. But this is what it may well be. How does one tell the difference between this expression of illness and one that is non-erotic?

As with Anastasia, the patient's presentation of a psychological problem seems to have a life of its own. If the analyst understands it, the patient seems unconsciously intent upon re-presenting it in slightly altered form. There seems to be an intelligence to this illness, as if it insisted upon remaining alive and attaching itself to analysis. In fact, it is a form of auto-erotic enclosure, castrating the other's phallus, now used as an internal self object within the private ongoing reveries of an unending transference addiction.

The borderline personality will seek turbulence as an end in itself, because a distressed state of mind is equivalent to the primary object, and will foster conflict with the analyst in order to feed off this object relation. The entrenched hysteric's suffering is more articulate and elaborate, like an erotic plant that grows in the light of the psychoanalytical space. In this frame of mind, the patient has no intention of 'co-operating with analysis' except to keep it going forever. If the patient is challenging, as entrenched hysterics inevitably are, he or she seeks to elucidate and materialise the analyst's interpretive skill, which is erotised. Even if, as with Anastasia, the analyst interprets that the patient intends for the analyst interpretively to penetrate the patient with his knowledge-phallus, the content of the interpretation itself never escapes the nature of its function: ironically, captured in this very content. The symptom – this suffering that invites the attention of the other – always seeks the penetrating other, finding in psychoanalysis an erotic life more than fulfilling in itself.

Many would argue that an Anastasia suffers a type of borderline dependency and would attend to her ego weakness as an explanation of her situation. Her attachment to her objects would be stressed, as would her inability to separate and individuate. These perspectives are not incorrect so far as they go, but they are incomplete, and do not attend to a most important detail. The patient's attenuation of pathology is an erotic expression, rooting itself in the analytical object. Each time this pathology is partly removed through interpretation, its intelligence is aimed at renewing the removed portion, so that this patient is particularly difficult to treat, since the unconscious motivation is directed towards the extension of the love relation.

Anastasia's mind is her sex object, as it conjures images and sensations that are auto-erotically pleasing. She can achieve a type of orgasm, spending herself in the tension between long spells of resistance and sudden bursts of self disclosure. The schizoid personality also uses the mind as an object, to replace the otherness of the other. Thinking about the other – only living as the schizoid's mental object – is preferable for the schizoid to relating to the other. The hysteric does not use the mind to eradicate experience of the other, but, instead, the mind is a sexual object-in-itself, one to be played with to the point of occasional insight orgasms. He or she invites the analyst into 'mind-fucking' interpretations that will sustain the analyst's phallic power and ensure the patient's position as pre-genital supplicant, dominated by the adult world.

Anastasia's ability to present herself as incompletely analysed by any analyst evoked clinical desire in the new analyst, who genuinely felt that the previous analysis had been incomplete and that further work was warranted. Hysterical desire, then, operates in the analyst's countertransference, functioning as his or her commitment to the patient's presumed analytical needs. To accomplish this tie, the analysand must falsify the prior analyses, diminishing them in order to lure the new analyst into the psychoanalytic romance.

This particular form of lying aims to eliminate, from both self awareness and the knowledge of the other, vital parts of the truth (or the story) that inconvenience the self's determination to adhere to the state of childlike dependency. The dynamic lack in the analysand – incompleteness as lure – is projected into the former analyses, which are seen as themselves incomplete. Accepting relocation of lack, the new analyst unwittingly takes part in a collusive projection, and so the process continues with no conclusion intended.

Certain hysterics become transference junkies. They find in the cosy erotism of psychoanalysis a state suited to a form of hysterical life: as the self lies alongside the erotic other, the absence of physical intimacy is itself continually exciting. Talking and talking the self to the analyst, the hysteric finds in speech not simply discharge; the analyst's voice becomes an erotic object for voice intercourse, each entering the other through the ear. This immaculate conception gives birth to many analytical children – the many turning points and insights, offspring of the intercourse.

The sexuality of psychoanalysis is used by the entrenched hysteric to eradicate any sexual life with an other in the real. Typically, these analysands enter analysis in their twenties and live within the transference for the duration of their pro-creative years; abandoning the search for an erotic partner until it is too late, they remain in analysis to grieve the loss of possibility. The fact that psychoanalysis itself has become the patient's symptom often seems to elude the analyst. Certainly, the idea that the analyst must impose a termination date in order to end the analysand's unconscious corruption of the analytical process and bring them into reality is too rarely considered.

It is rarely considered, of course, because the hysteric who is caught up in psychoanalysis as the symptom of hysteria often senses the possibility of termination well before it enters the analyst's mind and deepens his or her ailment. Indeed, it is not uncommon for hysterical psychosis to emerge as a final rebuff to any proposed separation. One can sympathise with the analyst who, finding himself or herself with a patient who seems lost in some fog, suffering from uncontrollable grief, barely able to speak, sometimes collapsing in public spaces, and worrying to friends, stops feeling that termination was a good idea. The analyst is likely to think that he or she has missed something, not realising that the arrival of the missing is the continual lure in the hysteric's claim upon the object.

One solution to the dilemma proposed by this form of transference is to do what Freud did in his treatment of the Wolf Man: to set a termination date some years ahead of time. The date as a reference point in the symbolic order takes on many meanings: the end of omnipotent transference claims; the limits of analysis; the end of life. The analyst brings the father into the analytical space and insists upon his effect. As the date approaches, the symbolic function now refers to the arrival of the real, and the hysteric must find a place in life that accepts all the endings that beset any self. If the duration of analysis before this termination phase has been ample – let's say four to six years – then the analysand's hysteric structure has benefited from the work of analysis. Remembering that entrenched hysterics insist on the preservation of illness, analysts nonetheless must set the date knowing that the patient will act out in ways determined to prove the analyst wrong. It probably helps if the analyst has actually had children and knows from experience what it is like to stand firm and insist on endings, even if this is sometimes in the face of the child's hysteria.

The analyst may also have to live with the real possibility that the patient will simply choose another analyst and sustain his or her entrenchment. But at the very least the analyst will have sustained the function of the father and brought the hysteric into meaningful contact with the real. Even if the patient seems to subvert this through further analysis, the analyst will not have colluded with such self-abuse, an important part of the analyst's status as an ongoing internal object in the patient's world.

However, psychoanalysts are often not in the best position to analyse the dynamic interminability of hysterical passion for psychoanalysis, as it is not uncommon for psychoanalysts to have entrenched *themselves* in excessively long psychoanalyses – ten to fifteen years – or multiple analyses that have them on the couch for decades. Can we say that in these analyses there has truly been an analysis of the analyst's transference to his or her analysis, as the custodian of psychoanalysis? I am not so sure. In such circumstances I cannot see how the psychoanalyst would be psychically equipped to analyse the hysterical analysand, as he would have converted psychoanalysis into a symptom of his or her own hysteria. Under what terms do psychoanalyses continue for decades? Certainly, only by turning a blind eye[1] to the failure that presents itself to both psychoanalyst and analysand.

Note

1   See John Steiner's book *Psychic Retreats*.

Chapter 13

Seduction and the therapist

Quentin is a psychologist who had an extensive practice looking after people with eating disorders and sexually dysfunctional clients. He read widely in the analytical literature, especially in the fields of self psychology, object relations and separation–individuation. He believed that most of his patients had been traumatised by faulty parenting in their childhoods and that the patient needed some form of transformation through a new type of empathy functioning in the clinical environment. He believed that the patients should be encouraged to express openly their feelings about anything that was bothering them; when they reported episodes from daily life to him he would invariably ask, 'And how does that leave you feeling?', whereupon his clients would open up certain floodgates of affect.

It seemed to those working with him or supervising him that many of his clients were indeed very 'damaged' and his open, friendly and compassionate stance was seen as appropriate. He would commonly sit on the couch with patients who were in distress and now and then ask them if they wanted to hold his hand or have his arm around them. Apparently, most did. And, apparently, that was the end of that.

Susie sought treatment with Quentin because she 'had no confidence' in herself and was distraught by a recent romantic rejection, which seemed to confirm to her that she was 'a loser'. In the months to follow she narrated a rather bleak picture of her childhood, mostly characterised by family moves that never seemed to work out for anyone, by the birth of four siblings who failed to nourish the parents, by the low self-esteem of the mother and the distant remove of the father. Susie was distraught during these tellings and was often in floods of tears.

Quentin was deeply moved by her account. He urged her to go with her feelings and she did. He asked her to elaborate on any of the particular details she seemed to be remembering and she did. He said she had no belief in herself because she had not been supported by either of her parents and he told her that therapy was a place where she could expect to have such support.

Quentin's practice was to issue the following message on his answering machine: 'Hello, this is Quentin X. I am sorry that I am not able to reach my phone right now. If you want to speak to me urgently, please call me on xxx. If this is an emergency please call ooo. Please leave any message of any length after you hear the tone.' With the very disturbed people he had in treatment he felt obliged to offer a proper treatment plan in which patients were given clear access to him. He pointed to the success of this plan by indicating that it was very common for his patients to call him and leave long messages on his machine, which he was quite sure functioned as a container for their anxieties.

It seemed to him quite appropriate to ask Susie if he could sit with her on her couch in order to hold her hand. She was deeply moved when he asked and told him that no one had ever shown such care for her in the past. Once she held his hand, however, she did not want to let go and each session she would ask if he would sit with her on the couch and just hold her hand. She brought a small teddy-bear from home and asked if she could leave it with Quentin, who agreed and stored it in a cabinet drawer labelled with the patient's first name. Again, this was standard practice as the cabinet had the names of other patients and their various deposited objects.

When Susie did not show up for one of her sessions, Quentin was quite surprised. There was no message on his machine. Nor did she return any phone calls. The following day, however, Quentin found a stranger in his waiting-room who passed him an envelope containing a subpoena. Susie was suing him for sexual molestation. The civil charge against him was not pursued, although a charge was brought against him by the state licensing board. He was censured for holding a patient's hand, which was regarded as provocative. Susie, whom he never saw again, did not take matters further.

In the aftermath of this episode, a shocked Quentin did not know what had happened to him. He was stunned by her allegation that he had sexually molested her and could not understand where it had come from. Perhaps, he mused, the mere fact of being touched in such a circumstance had de-repressed Susie's experience at the hands of an actual truly sexually molesting other. Had her father molested her, he wondered?

In reviewing his clinical notes for supervisory purposes, however, it became clear that Susie did indicate to him that she found contact with him sexually stimulating. For example, in the first hour she said that she found him to be 'the first man in my life who really understands me' and in subsequent hours many of her allusions were to the sexual content of the event. But Quentin had understood these references in what he regarded as 'self terms', as expressions of need and gratitude. It apparently never crossed his mind that the patient might have experienced sexual feelings for him or experienced the hand-holding as a sexual event.

The breakdown of a therapy like this is very common indeed. The reasons for its breakdown are also equally common. There is a collusion between the patient's reluctance to express sexual contents and the therapist's equal reluctance to bring it up. Indeed, more commonly than not, the patient is rebuffed when bringing up sexual feelings, which are often translated into the language of the self, or the language of affect, or the language of dependence. In effect, then, the sexual content is refused by the analyst and the patient and both seek a transcendent solution.

When the hysteric forms a florid erotic transference with an analyst, however, it presents unique problems.

Gerald, the senior vice-president of a medium-sized corporation, sought analysis in his mid-thirties after divorcing his wife, to whom he had been married for twelve years. It had been a tempestuous relationship, with his former wife often threatening to kill herself and enacting scene upon scene at home and in public, which put Gerald in the position of the sane, loyal and clearly admirably suffering partner. His marital problems had, he thought, consumed so much of his time and his energy that he wanted to understand how he got himself into such a mess and he wanted to reappraise his future.

However, within a few months of beginning analysis with his female analyst – who was his contemporary – he was disconcerted to discover that he found her more than attractive. Day after day he was preoccupied with her and now and then he alluded to his desires in sessions, but the analyst did not analyse these allusions and instead employed a neutral sexless language to discuss Gerald's 'self-empowerment issues'.

As time passed, he became truculent and very childlike, pleading for her empathy and understanding, as he said he now found life not worth living, and was deeply preoccupied with suicide. In each session he discussed his latest suicide fantasies. The analyst understood these preoccupations as expressions of his disappointment that he could not be the sole object of her attention, which she sensitively linked to his feelings that she was not attuned to his despair. She offered more sessions per week – which he accepted – and she was 'on call' when he would telephone her in particular states of distress.

In time, however, the analyst realised that she had failed to take up the patient's erotic transference, which had manifested itself very early in the analysis. She waited for him to allude to his desire in a session, which he did, and she said that she had failed to understand his expressions of passion, which must have left him feeling eradicated as a man, and now only like a defeated and worthless boy.

The patient was relieved by her understanding of this particular truth, and the severity of his despair, including the romance with suicide, abated. But the analyst was stunned by what followed next, as the patient launched into intensely sexual narratives session after session. Typically, he would enter the room and after lying down comment on how she looked. She was flushed or pensive or joyful or whatever psychic quality he thought he had seen, and he linked each of these states to her feelings toward him. She would be flushed because the physicality of his arrival had taken her by surprise. She was pensive because she was trying to figure out how to tell him she was in love with him. She was joyful because this was the last day she would sustain a professional relation to him and in a matter of moments would announce her love.

He noted not only what she wore, but told her how it hung on her body. How it accentuated her thighs, her breasts, her bottom or other parts of her body. He talked about what they would do after they married, what sort of house they would buy, what sorts of joint hobbies they would have, what holiday spots they would visit, which foreign languages they would study, what kinds of friends they would have.

He dreamed and associated to his dreams. He brought up issues from work which bothered him. He occasionally offered insights into his character, which he lamented as unfortunate. But even though there were these apparently neutral dimensions, he was hopelessly besotted by his analyst.

One might think, then, that his overt discussions of how he would make love to the analyst were in themselves particularly disconcerting. 'I am going to throw you down on the desk, spread your legs, and come into you like a wild stallion.' Or one might think that his erotic reveries, which gradually assumed a kind of narrative presence, were also countertransferentially disconcerting. 'I am thinking of your breasts . . . just your lovely breasts . . . they're all that's on my mind.' The analyst did feel, looking back, that she had failed adequately to speak up for Gerald's erotic states of mind, and as she was newly qualified she acknowledged that this was the first male patient who called upon her to discuss sexuality in such a frank and matter-of-fact way, but she did not find his transference either mentally invasive, offensive or, for that matter, erotic. She said that it was as if she was in the presence of someone caught up in an intense daydreaming. Without knowing it at the time, she had identified a male hysteric's erotic transference and distinguished it from a perverse erotic transference or a sexualisation of the transference communicated to the countertransference.

What Gerald brought to his analysis were previously unconscious sexual fantasies which had been repressed, although many of them had been acted out by his wife, who would talk about her sexual life in highly exhibitionistic ways. He had been 'the good boy' not just in relation to his wife, but for much of his life. His sexual life had averted the other and with his girlfriends and his wife he was a care-giver rather than a sexual partner. But for as long as he could recall, he had been a daydreamer and from adolescence throughout his adult life had had intensely erotic daydreams about imaginary and real people. For example, for three years he had intense erotic fantasies about the check-out woman in the lunch room of his corporation. He had never had a private conversation with her, but he always asked how she was doing and she always gave him a broad smile when she saw him. He would also glance over her way when picking up his lunch and she would return the glance in ways that assured him she was also preoccupied with him. When he approached her his heart would be pounding, he would sometimes blush and drop his change, and she too seemed flustered, but one day she was not at the counter and it took him weeks to ask after her, whereupon he discovered that she had moved to another city. Two weeks later he fell into a passionate romance with a secretary who worked for a colleague of his and whom he saw each day because she brought him his post.

When he transferred his auto-erotic reveries to his analyst he found the hysterical object of desire. Out of the abstinence of psychoanalysis, which forbids sexual intercourse between its participants, an unrequited love would allow Gerald to become a Petrarch to a Laura, addressing his love sonnets to the object of his passion. She is meant simply to listen, meant to be transported into his narrative, meant to live with him in the auto-erotic universe. For, as discussed in the early chapters of this book, this is where the hysteric's erotic life thrives in the daydream attached to the other. If the mother could not erotise the actual body of her infant, and if, furthermore, she was averse to celebration of her husband's sexuality and avoided acknowledgement of her children's genital identities, she was not sexually dead, but sexually shy, living her passions in her own private world of erotic reverie. In self-stimulating erotics, mother and self gently attach love to the other and split off the raw movement of sexuality, which can flourish in the deep privacy of the inner life. A flushed face. A startled cry. A step back in surprise. These are the signs of hidden desire.

In the present analytical situation the analyst is not meant to speak. She is meant to be a silent witness, not distinguishing her status as other from her position as object. The sight of her at the beginning of the hour is sufficient to promote many further sightings in the imaginary as the patient conjures her erotic being in his mind. If he speaks to the analyst as other, this is mere illusion. He is speaking out loud, celebrating a love life that is at that moment proceeding as it should. If he cries, demanding that she accede to his desires, spread her legs and let him make love to her, he does not want to hear back from the other; he is in possession of the object – as always in the universe of erotic reverie.

When Gerald's analyst did embark on analysis of the unconscious intentions of his desire, he was initially very upset. He returned to the state of mind of a petulant and suicidal self, in effect, warning the analyst that she was endangering the two of them by taking such risks with her speech. But she analysed this negative transference as his coercive effort to put the disruptiveness of sexuality into herself, to assign her blame for it, and to leave him a good, if once again battered and misunderstood, boy. In the two years following this change in her analytical focus, the patient revived his relation to his father, who had long been seen as cold and distant, but who now could be seen as his competitor whom he banished to the wilderness. His erotic reveries changed in their intensity, from near-orgasmic masturbations to mnemic events saturated with grief over losing the mother. The analyst's breasts, or bottom, or thighs were now like signs of lost objects, but increasingly he talked about work and different women whom he found interesting. When he realised that all his life he had been choosing auto-erotic sex objects rather than sex objects from the real, and when he could see that this was linked up with his wish to be a good boy rather than a sexual man, a strategy which imposed limits on his maturation and the realisation of adult ambitions, he found himself in a period of intensely meaningful struggle between these two vectors. In the end, he gave up the predominance of the auto-erotic universe and the mnemic erotics of the mother's body and found a real sex object in the world with whom he got on with his life.

Ultimately, Gerald was willing to 'talk about it' as well as to 'talk it'. In doing so, he contributed to the very basics of the psychoanalytic therapeutic for the hysteric: what Breuer and Freud (1893) accurately termed the 'talking cure'. By talking the erotic scenes, the imagery was transformed into speech, enabling the self to move from the maternal to the paternal order. Separated from the hallucinatory satisfactions of the imaginary (maternal) order, which give the illusion of a harmonious unity with one's objects, the self is now in the negotiated world of the symbolic order, where speech breaks the self into fragments derived from the unconscious.

Another patient.

Florence did not go gently into that kind of light. She selected her analyst after seeing him walking in the street. Although in many respects a good patient – describing her history in remarkably detailed and fine ways, contemplating her current domestic life situation, which was somewhat stressed, reporting and associating to her dreams – she very soon found her analyst's way of listening, thinking and talking 'delicious'. Although from a working-class family she had done well in her A-level exams, had attended one of the finest universities in England and went on to enter an accomplished profession. She was astute, interesting, reflective and in many respects an exceptional and attractive person.

But she found in her analyst a figure around whom she could conjure a wealth of erotic fantasies. Although she alluded to these scenes and, in response to analytical interpretation, would report them under duress, as the years passed the analyst surmised that they were increasing in their intensity and in their function.

Florence knew that she had suffered a type of maternal refusal; indeed, it continued into the present time. Although she was an only child, the mother was a self-absorbed woman who was immersed in her hobby – she collected garden gnomes – and the father was a remote man who seldom spoke except in well-worn and familiar clichés such as 'So Florence . . . how is work then?' The parents continued to live in their seaside bungalow, its front lawn populated by their 'real' family, a veritable village of gnomes, which they sold to fellow collectors. When Florence stayed with her family she felt an intense despair creeping over her.

As a child she had completely absorbed herself in romantic literature, which she continued through studying novels of the eighteenth and nineteenth centuries at university, and subsequently in her profession, which suited this kind of pre-occupation. She had had love relations, always beginning with great passion, only to be turned off with almost equal coldness, followed by periods of dehydrated discourse with her soon to be ex-lover. She would already have 'espied' another man in her surroundings and, unknown to her soon departing lover, would be absorbed with this new man.

Unfortunately, Florence succeeded in defeating the analysis of her hysteria, although she benefited from it in other respects. To the very end, she cultivated a type of delusional erotic transference, sustained by the unrequited-love structure of analysis and the privilege of silence. In this milieu her imaginary world took hold and flourished as it had not done in the presence of the other since early childhood. For Florence it was sufficient that she could love this proximate other intensely. She did not want to talk about it, for fear of losing the love relation. Instead, she kept it inside her, largely in her erotic musings whilst in the presence of the analyst.

Psychoanalysis does not dictate a patient's future. Florence's analyst accepted that she would refuse the dissipation of her love through talk and that she would continue to use the transference as food for love. He discussed this with her on innumerable occasions. Sometimes she would agree. Sometimes she would protest that her love was not transferential but real (he had never said it was not real). Sometimes she would say that she knew one day he would fall in love with her and she was not prepared to give him up. Sometimes she would say that she knew they would never be lovers in the true sense, but it did not matter, as she knew he loved her and she loved him. Sometimes she would say that he did not deserve to hear of her love, which to him was only the material of interpretation, whereas for her it was the substance of her soul. And sometimes she would ostensibly 'talk it', but this would consist of highly detailed descriptions of how she would like to make love to him.

Another psychoanalyst and another patient.

Jerome is a psychoanalyst practising in a small city, where he has developed a reputation as a gifted clinician and a thoughtful teacher. There are few psycho-analysts in his neck of the woods and virtually all those interested in analysis have at one time or another worked with him. Heather is a social worker who sought him out for analysis, as she felt that she was incapable of having a relation. She is an attractive woman who lives alone and is the same age as her analyst.

Jerome found her an immensely appealing patient and he reported to colleagues in a peer group that now and then he found her momentarily exciting, but other-wise he simply felt 'clinically significant'. He understood her to be a borderline patient who could not stand on her own feet because she lacked a profound sense of self and in time her increased dependence on him seemed to confirm her lack of a core sense of self. As she was also a mental-health worker, it seemed sensible to him now and then to give her professional articles he had read and found interesting. He told his group that he felt she needed partly to develop a sense of self through her own emerging professional self.

Within about three years Heather flowered. She transformed herself from an attractive, somewhat diffident woman to a stunningly dressed person and a passionate advocate of psychoanalysis. She praised her analyst to friends and colleagues, and indeed referred several patients to him, which he accepted with gratitude. Both analyst and patient felt that part of her development was a direct result of Jerome's encouragement to read papers, attend conferences and, indeed, to collaborate with him on book reviews. He knew this was somewhat unusual – as did his patient – but they discussed it and justified it on the grounds that she was being empowered through auxiliary ego work on the part of her analyst.

Heather's transference deepened and became deeply loving. She idealised her analyst, and told him that she was in love with him and would want to marry a man like him. The analyst accepted this as an expression of her new-found sense of self and believed that her love was essential to her personal evolution. When she became despondent because she could not marry him, Jerome often interpreted that, although marriage was not a possibility, she could retain some connection with him after the end of analysis, because they would be colleagues together.

After the end of analysis, Heather would argue that she had in fact conveyed to Jerome that she felt more than just platonic love for him, that she felt herself in a state of constant arousal every time she saw him. But Jerome seemed 'disinterested', always interpreting any of these feelings as indications of her ability to love, which was an important part of her development into adult life. When Jerome discussed this with his colleagues he said that he thought she had a kind of borderline sexual interest in him, which he understood as passing part-object sexualisations that were failed constituents of a more ego-integrative attitude towards him. He said he felt it was important to accept her sexualisations without exploratory comment, so that they could be transformed into higher-level affective and intellectual sentiments, which would serve her development.

After six years of analysis they seemed to many to be a hard-working analytical couple, as the patient's life improved in her personal demeanour, her economic well-being and her professional circumstances. They seemed colleague-like. It did not seem out of context, therefore, for Jerome to encourage Heather to attend a conference with him, and to travel with him – roughly an eight-hour car journey. Heather took it as yet another confirmation of her analyst's belief in her. Indeed, the journey proceeded seemingly innocuously; they both presented papers, and then drove back.

Unfortunately, this psychoanalyst, whose own personal analysis and training had not been adequate, did not appreciate that he was colluding with an hysterical analysand's erotisation of the transference. More regrettably, the analysand did not have an analyst whose skill was equal to her needs for analytical comprehension of her neurosis. During the car ride, Heather wore a sexually revealing outfit that the analyst found exciting. On the return journey she blurted out to him that she wanted him to make mad passionate love to her. He rebuffed her suggestions and told her that they would never have that kind of relationship, although he was to tell his peer group that in fact he found her incredibly exciting and had thought about 'fucking her brains out' at the conference.

Heather's rage at the analyst's refusal was considerable and she reported him to his psychological association for malpractice. (Fortunately for Jerome, he had been in a peer group reporting on this case for many years, so he could draw on those colleagues to report this case to his own association, which censured him – for inappropriate contact with a patient, by attending a conference together, etc. – but did not remove his licence.) When he sought further consultation on this case and reviewed his notes, it was not difficult for the consultant to see that the analyst had consistently declined to speak to the patient's expression of erotic interest in him. Indeed, he had continually transformed it into the language of 'need' or into affective references, so if the patient had said 'I have this wish to just be with you and to feel your body', he would reply, 'The baby-you wishes to be close to mother-me.' The patient would frequently cry in response, which he took to be confirmation of his interpretations, but it was pointed out to him that these were more likely to be tears of loss, as he had not actually comprehended her communication and, furthermore, that by crying she could gain some small orgasmic-like relief from the tension that she experienced.

It was painful to see how the analysand's erotic intensities had not only been consciously misunderstood by the analyst, but also – at least in part – unconsciously colluded with: by exchanging gifts and professional engagements, the analysand was allowed to feel that there was a promise of symbolic sexual intimacy. To be sure, her sexuality was in fore pleasure alone, but that only made the analyst's inadequacy all the more unfortunate. For it was in the cycle of arousal and deferral, arousal and deferral, that the patient found her erotism establishing itself. She convinced herself that her analyst loved her but was prevented by professional decorum from saying so; therefore when he took her for the drive in the car, she viewed this as his only way of getting the object of desire. The drive to the conference, during which they discussed their lives, was like some strange kind of dream. Although in the past it had been hurtful to her to hear Jerome refer to his wife and his children, she knew now that passing references to them were merely signs of what a wonderfully devoted man he was. He was leaving it to her to breach his honour. She would have to sweep him off his feet. She knew that if she was brave enough to declare her passion, he would give in and they would marry.

This was not a new belief; it had been growing in intensity for well over a year. In sessions she took his refusals to discuss her sexuality more explicitly as the result of shyness, all the more exciting for her, as she could see in him her former self. She was amused that she seemed to be gaining in confidence in an important area of life, whilst he seemed less capable, but she could see that he did indeed look at her with occasional flashes of clear sexual interest.

In the three months leading up to the conference, knowing they would travel together, she was almost beside herself. Out of respect for his sense of boundaries she did not press her case in the sessions. She did bring him flowers, books and objects for his office, and she did so gracefully and with such skill that, although he said she should not do this, she was able to overpower him. In her mind, she was now looking after him and establishing something of a home in the consulting room. But the moment when they were to 'break it to one another' would have to be in the car; that was why he had accepted her suggestion to travel together.

Heather subsequently alleged that Jerome had engaged her in many physical encounters – from hugging and hand-holding to kissing – that constituted his sexual attack on herself. He was to counter-argue that he hugged her to console her during deep borderline regressions, that he did hold her hand when she was also in states of deep distress, and that he never kissed her on the mouth, but did kiss her on the forehead, in what he took to be a parental manner, simply to confirm to her that she was loved by an other.

It is useful to consider the difference between the schizoid and hysteric erotic transferences. Starved of an actual relation to the alive other – incarcerated in the mental house-arrest of schizoid detachment – the schizoid sexualises the erotic transference and is oftentimes quite dramatically in love. But the hallmark of schizoid erotics is a surprising shock that becomes a kind of celebrated laboratorial surprise. 'My God, look what I feel about you', he or she extols, often in a manic way. Both schizoids and hysterics exhibit their desire, but whereas the schizoid's love is in the laboratory, the hysteric's is in the theatre. The schizoid is observant like the hysteric – both are watching their desire – but the schizoid is obsessed with his or her sexualised inner objects (and the analyst in the transference), whereas the hysteric watches the effect of his or her desire upon the other. The hysteric's witness is always in the place of the third object. The schizoid derives no such secondary gain from his or her anguish; he or she genuinely does not know what to do with this love. The hysteric derives unending secondary gain from his or her pain, which becomes a collateral object of desire. The schizoid experiences a resourceless state, the hysteric feels curiously more powerful.

The schizoid patient who erotises the transference can decompensate into delusional psychosis. If hospital becomes necessary he or she will be in a closed unit and under heavy sedation. The hysteric can apparently be every bit as mad-in-love, but at the hospital always becomes calm and lucid, and can walk out of the mad scene as if nothing had happened. The schizoid in love cannot do this.

The schizoid seeks a cure by talking to the other about the other's status as his or her internal object. But this talking is a magical act, as the schizoid seeks to speak only to the internal object; ultimately, a defiance of the other and the play of interrelating. The hysteric also talks a lot, as we know, seeking to capture the analyst in an inner world of sorts: the hysteric's theatre. Hysterical auto-erotism is a type of schizoid manoeuvre, replacing self–other engagement with the theatre of the internal world. But hysteria involves a well-known course of erotic manage-ment, one that finds in repression, displacement, indifference and conversion the familiar shape of desire. It gives to this auto-erotism a route for sexuality, and the hysteric is always moving his or her objects through a known course of events. Finding an other to love, experiencing understanding and empathic recognition, the schizoid's love of the analyst is an overwhelming emotional experience that threatens the schizoid's psychic economy. His or her effort to re-internalise the other – to convert the other to object alone – follows the path of familiar detachment; yet, owing to the force of love in the transference, it will not work.

Even though hysterical scopophilia drives the hysteric's observation of his or her own mad love affairs, and even though the erotic transference courses through the hysteric's body opera as possession by primal scene, the hysteric in sexual love aims to be rid of the disturbance of instinctual life. The analyst's refusal to reciprocate the erotic expression becomes the basis of a new erotism: the excitement of self-sacrifice. Here in his or her abstinence the analyst unwittingly becomes the ideal sex object, the one who refuses to allow sex to ruin the relationship. The analyst's function is irresistible. What the hysteric passes off as grief stricken by frustration is an exaggerated auto-erotic mirroring of the self-sacrifice of the analyst. To keep this scene going, the hysteric, ironically, has no choice but to sustain the demand for sexuality.

Chapter 14

The last chapter

We come now to the end of this study of hysteria – surely the most complex character in psychoanalytic theory – faced with bringing some of the main points of the thirteen previous chapters into a single picture. What do we have?

The hysteric elects to perpetuate a child innocent as the core self, endeavouring to be the ideal boy or girl throughout a lifetime. He or she is always performing this child through the body of the adult, impishly undermining the ostensible effect of the biological maturation of the self. He or she is the 'child within' who castrates the self's achievements in the real by periodic uprisings that shed the self of the accoutrements of accomplishment. This psychic position is to serve as the fountain of youth, driving off ageing and death, and conferring upon the hysterical character a sense of immortality.

The hysteric asks fellow innocents for communion, passing back and forth memories, identities and new-found ideas, as ghosts in a character seance that transmit and receive all internal objects in impressionistic and impressionable exchanges. These intense communications, like water purifiers, cleanse the self of the impurities of reality by constant reprocessing of the news of the day. Talking and talking and talking the self to the other (or listening and listening and listening) serves up the occasional hot topic that drives the speech cathexes.

To identify with and represent the other's internal objects is the hysteric's passion, easily satisfied by reading books or watching films, where the self enjoys the illusion of secret access to the other's imaginary. Here, as an insider, the hysteric succumbs to deep reverie, becoming the objects he or she reads or sees, taking them off afterwards and re-experiencing them in tellings to the other. In intimate relations the hysteric demands endless access to the other's internal world. 'What are you thinking about?' 'You must tell me what you thought about the film . . . in great detail!' These demands become the daily territorial song of the hysteric, who enters the other's imaginary, trying out the other's introjects for size, seizing or casting some off, re-dressing the self in the other's internal garments, intended to mirror the other to himself or herself. Hysterics scrutinise the other in disconcerting ways, penetrating a resistant other with critical gaze, aiming to dislodge inner objects like knocking fruit down from a tree. The hysteric would seem to enjoy excoriating the other with deconstructive precision, but unlike the paranoid – who projects the self into the other and then feels haunted by the other's presumed hostile response – the hysteric's hostility is an act of identification with a powerful superego, aiming to gain scopophilic access through its lofty position. The Carmelite mood of the hysteric's use of sexual politics affects a furrowed brow to inspire confessional sexual exhibitionism in the other, forming a parasitic critique that feeds off the other's crimes and misdemeanours.

Constantly disavowing his or her body, the hysteric apologises for carnal impositions, attacking his or her sexuality by refusing to his or her instincts gratification through the other. The other, too, is asked to renounce carnal intent, from which spiritual currency is coined that will pave the way for both partners to enter a more divine household. The hysteric lives this family romance to the hilt, always implying that he or she is only on loan to the material world, for at a future date the hysteric will be called forth by his or her heavenly parents to return to the holy family from which he or she originates. It was not only Jesus who left the earthly world to join his holy family; he paved a road walked by all hysterics, who renounce carnal interests to testify to their nobler existence.

Unsurprisingly, hysterics are intensely ambivalent about imagining and delivering genital sexuality, as they believe that it is sinful and that they will lose their innocence. The great moments of the body in the self's life – the sexual epiphanies of the 3-year-old and the 13-year-old – make the body a type of villain for hysterics. When they repress their repudiated sexual mental contents, it is fitting that they are converted into a body ailment to which they seem blithely indifferent: the body, agent of their demise, shall in turn suffer pain and 'unlove'.

The hysteric not only treats the body with contempt, but transcends carnality and the everyday, aiming to find a self and its others that inhabit a higher, spiritual realm of being. Body debasement is, in fact, the admission ticket to this region, where they shall find similar souls, sharing non-corporeal lusts. In this realm they will meet with their first other: the god who brought them into existence, the mother who communicated love of their souls and disgust with their sexual interests.

It is not by virtue of the maternal position, however, that the hysteric feels obliged to join the maternal imaginary; the mother remains the source of an unanswered question, seemingly holding the clue to the most powerful answers about being and existence. What does it mean, asks the unconscious, that she finds in the carnal the source of all evil? The hysteric cannot move away from this question.

The power of the question seems reaffirmed by the body's effect on the mind, particularly in adolescence, when once again instincts seem to drive the self away from more spiritual communications with others. Where have all the boys and girls gone? Gone to fucking hell, the hysteric might reply.

Hysterics decline psychic entry into the actual sexual universe, preferring instead to appropriate sexual discourse and use it in place of the real. They may, ironically enough, prove great talkers about the sexual, and not uncommonly prefer in moments of sexual possibility to talk about it rather than to do it. Indeed, the move to sexual engagement seems defiling: it is best left in the realms of the imaginary.

Although the mother regarded the genitalia with disgust, she consecrated the infant's body with her repressed and displaced excitations, as the other erogenous areas – ears, feet, head – became erotic objects. The hysteric is sexualised along the surface of the body and wears the ornaments of this erotism quite well, while sexual intercourse is not part of surface sex. While the normal person finds the surfaces moving the self towards increasing genital excitation and demand, the hysteric finds this sliding towards the genital an unwelcome slope and cools the self off with abrupt cessations of sexual exchange. While others find the genital demand moving both lovers towards the sense of mutual orgasm, a strange blend of the body's knowledge and the mind's ecstatic submission, the hysteric imagines the genital moment to be a desecration of the self's purity. Orgasm with the other, for the hysteric, would have to serve a higher purpose, allowing for its immediate transport into transcendent realms, such as thinking of intercourse serving the armies of Jesus, or bringing a child into the world, or pleasing the partner's wish for it.

This is not to say, however, that the hysteric does not have sexual desires and does not seek sexual orgasm. Through an act of splitting, the hysteric seeks to remain a sexual innocent whilst relieving itself of its excitations in fantasy. Auto-erotic sexuality seems permissible, even if the content of the fantasies suggests sexual relations to the other. Auto-erotic sexuality is private, tucked away, hidden from the other. It is willingly embraced as failed sexuality, finding in the limitations of auto-erotism refuge from the desecratory world of sexual intercourse. The impotent man and the sexually frigid woman are relieved to confess their problems to the other as they are then free to return to their auto-erotic enclaves, where they shall not be troubled by the sexual expectation of the other.

The auto-erotic sex object provides hysterics with all that they need. They do not consciously know, of course, that this object is the token of their mother's love; that in this derivative of thumb-sucking they find maternal erotism, unsullied by subsequent libidinal arrivals: anal, phallic, and so forth. They do not know that declining the invitation of the sexual other keeps them within the psychic zone of the infantile, resident in the maternal order, where both are meant to give up sex with any other, except within oneself. Sex within oneself, thumb for breast, permits hysterics to remain sexually excited yet never troubled by the demands of sexuality.

The hysteric forms an ambivalent relation to the father, who is associated with the intrusive demands of sexuality. He is to be rejected. But, ironically, the hysteric's refusal of the father constitutes part of the feature of the father: refused, the refusing, the no-figure. When the hysteric says 'no' to the father, he or she unconsciously celebrates the father as the one who says 'no', and, although in vigorous opposition to this figure, the father is hugely important in maintaining the hysteric's sanity. In Lacan's scheme of things, the hysteric has bound the imaginary by the symbolic order, has allowed the name of the father to subjugate the mother, but I think he or she has done it in the hysterical manner. That is, the hysteric has insisted that the name of the father be a 'no-no': a double 'no' in which the child says 'no' to the father's 'no', but celebrates the two noes.

The hysteric's echo of the paternal 'no' is charming. 'No' is seduced into an imaginary game of saying 'no' for its own sake; in the play of repetition, the hysteric creates a 'no'-theatre to exist alongside the enunciative performance of all the other schemes of life. The performance can be openly charming, as in the precocious vector of certain hysterias, meeting the future before it has opened in the present, and trouncing it with past considerations – or it can be alarming, as in the ascetic hysteric's embodiment of 'no': the severity of anorexia being the contemporary form.

The ascetic hysteric reflects the work of a type of death drive, one that mirrors maternal decathexis of the child's sexuality. Out of this decathexis the hysterical child finds maternal erotism, which seeks refuge from the other in the still posture of the statue body, frozen in time and space. As the ascetic hysteric identifies with a kind of ice mother, he or she also identifies with the mother's freezing of her sexuality, casting a strange glow on this person in adult life. The ascetic hysteric has sexualised virtue, deriving from abstinence a curious reflective pleasure, yet one which is always dynamically linked to the potential eruption of sexual pulsion and repulsion. This death drive, then, finds its energy in the libido of anti-cathexis; its passion is derived from the charge of withdrawal from the object of potential investment. Like the force of a 'backwater wave' – the wave that is sent back to sea by the reshaping curvature of the beach – it suggests a movement that will continue along its own course, but, unlike the backwater wave, the hysteric's anti-cathexes indicate a pure logic of systematic destruction of the self's sexual waves.

Freud argued that the state of absent-mindedness, which is a feature of repression, owes its existence to the loss of consciousness deriving from orgasm, especially auto-erotic ecstasy. Out of this type of withdrawal, then – the little death of orgasm – a principle is generated for the hysteric, in which the self will apply the pleasures of little deaths, one piling upon another, as the self retreats into death orgasm. Death-drive hysteria is unique, not following the course of the death instinct in the more severe pathologies. The hysteric has romanced death, just as he or she has charmed the father, finding in the art of absence – the mother's departure to begin with – the tease of death partings, then finding in little orgasms the echo of all losses of consciousness that seem strangely blissful.

The anorectic's erotism is his or her pleasure in the small deaths of the anti-ingestions. Where food was to have been there shall death libido be. Whether it is the refusal of food in the mouth, the refusal of the penis in the vagina, or (for the males) the refusal of an erection, the hysteric's counter-erotism is in the bliss of self-destruction. The anorectic's indifference to the body is an unconscious celebration of death, death now charmed out of its customary work – attacking the population at appropriate stages in biological time, through the usual illnesses – and appearing much too early in the real, yet forced to this prematurity by the romantic omnipotence of the anorectic. Friends, lovers and relations all witness the hysteric's relentless deterioration, feeling helpless to intervene, each long since seduced by the anorectic's child innocence. Talking to a saint about the body is hard work; and the saint's smile is so sweetly disarming.

The hysteric invites the other's seduction, and certainly many a person tries every trick in the trade to lure him or her back to life. But as the hysteric believes that human seduction is sad compensation for the failure of primary erotic love, he or she seduces the other's seduction into a type of gaze – 'Now look into my mirror and see how I transform your efforts into wonderful elaboration' – which removes each from the realm of real engagement on to a stage to perform a part each knows only too well. Both are meant to be captured by the other's internal world. Even though the hysteric acts out, often involving others in a kind of ongoing event, such enactments are always vested with auto-erotic libido – onanistic passions, daydreams operating under the cloak of apparent real relations. This is why the hysteric can suddenly leave off an intense involvement with people – either a scene at a convention or party, or a sequence of emotionally significant engagements with another person – leaving the other rather bewildered, as it had seemed so promising. To the hysteric, these encounters were only ever daydreams practised in reality upon actual others, who were to be seduced into intersubjective repressions: the exchanged mental contents disappear into ether, the hysterical surprise upon confrontation – 'oooh?' – a *petite mort* of meaning. In this surprise is the new-found libido of repression, functioning to drive each participant into self musings, wandering about in separate internal worlds and re-imagining what has just taken place in reality.

In sexual intercourse the hysteric's sex object is internal only, and the sexual other is engaged as a masturbation partner who shall screen carnal contents, which verge on guided imaginings. The hysteric's 'oh' – not the sign of 'O' which Bion gives to infinity, but the disappearance of the self into affinity – is pre-emptive orgasm, often occurring when the other announces sexual intention too boldly. 'Oh. Oh. Oh . . . I didn't realise . . .' 'Oh . . .' sounds the hysteric orgasm, disappearing through repression of sexual contents, into the bliss of renunciation.

The normal person finds in love-making a deep memory of intelligent erotics in the body response, initiation and handling – the love-making – of the other and this moment-in-the-real is deeply pleasurable, eradicating the fantasy objects as competitors. The normal individual finds the actual, not spectral body, of the lover in the real, deeply connective to the erotic drive. Such sexuality emerges from the core of one's being, derived from the love-making of mother and infant that inspires the erotic development of self. Not making love from the core, by contrast, the hysteric feels lost and alienated from this experience, in part because although the core is not felt, its absence at the moment of fulfilment is registered, and this becomes a disturbing presence. The hysteric's 'oh' transforms this loss into the superficial libido of surprise, which in turn announces the immanent pleasure of anti-cathexis as the hysteric prepares to beat a retreat into auto-erotic reverie.

In the fairy-tale world of hysterical fantasy there are love scenes and there are erotic objects. For every pulsion there is not a repulsion, but a transpulsion, as the hysteric's instinct finds objects that discharge the excitation upward into divine space. As the body is spent in its imaginings, the orgasm takes the form of the soul ascending towards heaven, whilst the body is left behind as a momentarily spent vessel. One of the functions of hysterical auto-erotism is to save the self for the imagined arrival of the divine. Through an act of dissociation the hysteric is only on erotic loan to any actual other who passes by. But such loans can act as toxic forms of promiscuity, the sexually gratified and gratifying self an exorcism of libido, violently ridding the hysteric of sexuality in order to return to purity and the virginal self's traditional place as self-in-waiting. One patient ended years of sexual isolation by sleeping with six men in one evening, a bizarre event in which she sought and received rape from a male group, but to which she lodged no objection – as they had sexually exploited her she was left paradoxically sated yet virginal: the rape was of their making, not hers. The idea that she should no longer engage the sexual other was obviously very inviting, and more than a few of her friends believed she would never sleep with men again.

Hysterical promiscuity uses an other who is always not-the-right-one, and is therefore expendable. But expendability is exciting, as it is a call to the instinct to use the object solely to discharge the self of the drive, allowing the hysteric to return to rest and sleep, the Sleeping Beauty of death.

There is always a question over whether the self should waste its eros with the not-the-right-one, as each time the self feels potential disqualification. This fosters a stop-and-go ambivalence in love-making, since this repetition neatly serves an exonerative function. The hysteric demonstrates the struggle. If he or she proceeds, it is because the hysteric is overcome by the demand of the other, who, witness to this frustration, steps in with a separate urgency. If the other refuses to participate in this exoneration, the hysteric becomes cold and enraged – not out of frustration, but because the self is then suspended in sexual foreplay, unable to conclude and thus allow exorcism to occur. Refused by the other, the hysteric is left stained by his or her own instinct, which is felt to be a mark against the self.

The hysteric often approaches any sexual other through identificatory compliance, a form of seduction in which the self assumes momentary blankness, or openness, ready to be the other's sex dream come to life. As the infant's sexuality was cosseted by the maternal imaginary, the hysteric assumes that his or her sexual meaning for the other is deeply held in the other's imaginary. So the hysteric says, 'I am whom you desire, your dream come true.' The other's approach is assumed to be equally auto-erotic, which is also enticing. In the hours or minutes before love-making the hysteric treasures the blanking of the self as sex offering. If the other also assumes this position then both express innocence or naivety as the foreplay.

The hysteric bears a distracted look during the day, so often lost in daydreams. Here he or she can be a hero, a great lover, an admired figure. In the daydream he or she meets ideal others engaged in the commerce of pure pleasure unsullied by the flesh of reality. The hysteric extends the realm of the daydream to a daydream consciousness, a type of perception that accepts daily realities only if they can be consecrated with daydream libido. An assistant at the check-out counter of the supermarket, a mother and child walking along the street, a newspaper article about a promising violinist, a telephone chat with a good friend – these bring not only warm smiles to the hysteric's face, they are cathexis centres, wells of good-breast feelings that over-privilege these moments, now to generate daydreams derived from these 'spots of time'. If the non-hysteric cultivates the psychic intensities of the day, to be dreamed – for better or worse – at night, the hysteric seeks to pre-empt the arbitrary power of dream life with the guided imaginings of the daydream. The day is to deliver to the self a plenitude of daydream orgasms, as the self takes its ecstasy from the auto-erotic base of moments that please the self.

Hysteric lovers-to-be may meet up for a film, stumble into rationalised need to visit one lover's flat, make tea in the kitchen, bump into one another like two internal objects cut loose, giddy with the oddity of their release into the real. They giggle a lot, and then talk and talk and talk. They may talk through the night. Other than the occasional collision there is no sexual touching. This would spoil the foreplay, the mutual presentation of innocence.

All the while, however, like a Christmas tree with flashing lights, each feels the charge of erotogenic zones over the body from time to time, in polymorphous excitation. A kiss, a move toward intercourse, would prematurely bind the pleasures of auto-erotic movement – the charging of the body by the absence of touch. Indeed, the hysteric feels deeply bonded to an other who reciprocates, as this encounter fulfils the earliest terms of the hysteric's love relation to the other.

Often enough the lovers-to-be do not have intercourse. Having spent themselves in speech – a dialogic avenue – they retire to separate dwellings, perhaps to meet again. The lingering questions – 'Does she desire me?'; 'Do I desire her?' – may verge on despair, carrying the child's forlorn feeling that he might not be the object of maternal desire after all. Further, if they had 'gotten into it' would she really have been to his taste? But the meeting was innocent, nothing did happen, there is no cause to feel sexually rejected or sexually rejecting, and the self may collect the imagery of the other in the erotism of *Nachträglichkeit*, the sexuality of afterwardness when the hysteric is made love to by a mnemic object.

If these lovers-to-be do make love, it arrives as a sudden violation of the real by the instinct. In the kitchen making tea, the one suddenly lunges for the other and they crash into one another, moving towards blind fucking. They have not seen it coming. They have not actually given time to, and therefore not seen, the erotic foreplay. They tear off clothes, jump into bed under the covers of darkness, and are ravaged by sex.

The hysteric intends it to be this way, if it is to be at all. The self is to be raped by the instinct. It is to disrupt and very possibly ruin the nascent relationship. After intercourse there may be a quick departure followed by assurances of a meeting in a few days' time. But that may be the end of it. Or they may promise that henceforth they should just be friends. It would only 'complicate matters' to do this. It seems easy enough to sacrifice sex to a higher purpose.

If they become a couple, establish a relationship and marry, they do so consenting that their love-making arrives when the instinct overwhelms their daily life as cohabiting innocents. They may apply their auto-erotic reveries to this occasion, making love to an ideal figure who is always absent. This absence is the mother, who shall preside from a distance over the self's sexuality, her absence nullifying immediate genital promise just as this refusal excites the total body that stands in for genital binding. Applying this scenario to the other, the hysteric may approach known likely sex encounters with auto-erotic elaboration. Yet love-making will usually be stereotypical (if elaborate) and often abrupt, almost violent in its comings and goings, leaving both wondering if the relation can survive this kind of disruption.

Hysterics carry a sense that they have cheated the lover. They have not opened their eyes to see the other's body. They are unfamiliar with the other's erotogenic preferences. They are non-communicative about their own erotogenic preferences. They are not interested in succumbing to the sexual logic of intercourse, following as it could the ineluctable future of orgasm that seems to be always in the present, seducing the self and other towards bliss in the future. The ecstasy of the body's 'not yet, not yet' is erotic promise of the future that rests inside the body's knowledge, carrying lovers to bliss. The hysteric knows little of this future – indeed, as always, he or she prefers suspension in the innocent's present as time out from the demands of the body and its imaginary consequence to human relations.

Freud was the first psychoanalyst to compare hysteria and perversion, a complex and possibly endless dialogue of two sexualities. Like the hysteric, the pervert is caught up in a form of auto-erotism. He or she is overwhelmingly occupied at times by an erotic fantasy that will need to be discharged. Like the hysteric, he or she may feel alienated by the instinct, sharing with the hysteric a paradoxical sense of personal innocence in the midst of overt, often bizarrely extensive, sexual practices. Both succumb to differing types of daydreaming. The hysteric is almost always somewhere else in his or her mind than where he or she is in reality. The somewhere else disincarnates the self, removing it from the labour of embodied existentiality. The hysteric is at play in his or her mind, only on loan to reality. The pervert is also often dissociated from the real, yet, whilst the hysteric's fantasies, if bordering on the sexual, involve romantic whole-object relations sacrificed to his or her destiny as a pure innocent (self-cancellation is orgasm of a sort), the pervert is driven by an erotic scene that is fragmented and, in its movement towards realisation, fragmenting to the self who would contain it.

The hysteric walking along the street caught up in one of countless daydreams and the pervert cruising for a sex object are semi-fugal beings, dissociated from reality. Under different spells, both are elsewhere. However, whilst the hysteric is innocent because blind to sexuality, the pervert is the sexual expert, presumed master of the instinct. For every psychic unit of alienation from his or her sexual fantasies the pervert conjures two units of anti-alienation, seeking to become a champion of his or her sexuality. If the hysteric seeks a fellow innocent to tantalise the self's polymorphous erotogeneity, yet be blind to it all as the way to see, the pervert seeks a fellow practitioner in the fine art of sexual technique. Whilst the hysteric shares sexual blankness with the other, the pervert shares sexual contents. Whilst the hysteric collects sex objects during the day to enjoy auto-erotic reveries in privacy, the pervert reverses the procedure and tries to export internal scenes into the real. The hysteric's auto-erotism is only slightly libidinal, as the collected objects are ideals, exciting as seemingly pure forms of sexiness or beauty in the other. They may be employed for self-stimulation, but otherwise they are figures in a kind of sexual church known for its sacrifice of sexuality to the gods. The pervert's auto-erotism seems overwhelmingly pre-ordained, specific and demanding. A self that only seeks an other with a leather glove on the left hand, wearing black leather boots, and holding a musical instrument in the right hand employed to strike the self repeatedly on the knee, is in no doubt about his or her preoccupation with the sexual.

The pervert feels that there is no boundary between his or her inner sexual life and the real. Indeed, as the pervert is seeking a black leather other or a boy or a woman wearing a hat, he or she is forced into reality to find such objects, which, as they always exist in the real, cumulatively erodes the boundary between psychic preoccupations and actions in the real. The pervert walking in the real is always on the prowl and when he or she sees an other wearing black leather or a boy or a woman wearing a hat, the pervert experiences a simultaneous double valence: from the instinct to the object, from the object to the instinct. This strange harmony gives the pervert an illusion of omniscience, as the world seems to constantly serve up exact objects of desire.

To enter the perverse zone – a disco of perverts, for example, where the others are regaled in highly specific sex costumes – is to encounter in the real a ready-made object for the instinct: it is as if the self's instinct ordered its objects before birth and only ever needed to search the environment for the delivery department. Perverse familiarity is entirely objective and programmatic; certain objects are sought and known means of object use come with instructions. The hysteric seeks the non-sexual dimensions of the other, refusing reduction to the sexual, insisting upon expansion to the transcendent or mental self-sacrifice in the interests of higher forms of love. The great literature of the pervert – de Sade, Sacher-Masoch – aspires to aesthetic and transcendent interests but as split-off falsifications of what is taking place in the real. In fact, the pervert is only interested in the other as a part sex object, seeing the other's leather or young body or hat and finding in this fragment (or token) the sole object of desire. Whilst the hysteric would gaze elsewhere, like Princess Diana's sidelong glance, the pervert stares directly – eyes wide open – at the other's sex thing.

The pervert and hysteric reverse one another, yet they share a common bond: conflict with sexuality preoccupies each with the sexual. Yet, whilst the pervert must have the other and enact the sexual, the hysteric must avoid the other and hide the sexual.

What makes the normal different from the pervert is that the normal meets a particular man or woman who is found to be intrinsically sexually attractive – his or her physical nature and personality are experienced as delightful. The pervert has a pre-arranged erotic meeting with the sex object. When meeting the other, the pervert psychically applies this object on to the other, or finds an other with a similarly predetermined sex scene that is applied.

The normal elaborates the idiom of the other through love, deriving fantasy material from play with the other. The hysteric seeks others as masturbation material and applies a masturbation fantasy to the other. He or she shies away from sexual encounters and uses repression as an erotic act. The pervert is driven compulsively by the sexual to the erotic place, which is sought before the other: literally and psychologically. The meeting or collision with the other is as important as the found other itself.

The normal unconsciously appreciates and erotically mirrors the love other, leading to a deeper form of unconscious communication. A deep sexual hunger is aroused and comes out of this meeting with the other. Sexuality and erotism, then, seem to derive from the arrival of the specific other and love is the predominant state of mind. Anxiety and alienation, meanwhile, are the predominant states of mind of the pervert, whereas dissociation and repulsion are the prevailing constituents of the hysterical frame of mind.

The mother of the hysteric ordinarily loves her infant's being, but is repelled by the infant's sexuality. The mother of the pervert either characterologically or circumstantially becomes emotionally cold towards her infant's being, but can be excited by the child's sexuality. The hysteric mother's abstention from sexual celebrations of her child's self, paradoxically, invites the child's unconscious search for this mother's desire, which always seems tantalisingly close to a transforming realisation. The hysteric is an optimist, feeling that his or her sexual petrifaction is momentary; good news is on the horizon. The mother will come round at last. The pervert mother expresses brief glimpses of violent excitation towards the child, providing near-death sensations, leaving the child disinclined to imagine her inner world. If she is, for example, circumstantially depressed – owing to the loss of a loved one, a disturbing move or the after-effects of birth itself – then her occasional libidinalisation of her infant's body, set against an otherwise deadened form of being, shocks the infant out of his or her state of nothingness by exploitation of the infant's instinct life, which seems to be evoked by the shocking arrival of something from the real. The pervert is a deep pessimist who feels that this mother, if transformed, would kill her child with overwhelmingly impersonal excitation. Maternal intervention shocks the infant, jolting him or her into a frozen and detached isolation, yet rousing the child's sensorium in a rush of anxiety that is linked unconsciously with maternal cathexis of his or her sexuality. These two excitations – the one roused by maternal intervention in the first place, the other by her cathexis of the child's body – are separate actions of the mother that become linked only by the child, who then combines the state of shock and the state of excitation into one psychic structure.

The pervert, initially victim of what feels like near-death experience, transforms such passivity into perverse activity, playing differing forms of death games with sexual partners. Whether perverts are bound and beaten, whether they beat the other, whether they are verbally dominated by an abusive other, whether they take pleasure in urinating on their object, or whether they use a fetish for intercourse, perverts portray themselves as masters of both their instincts and the otherwise coincidental arrival of the other. Wherever the other is found – in a bar, a toilet, or a club – the accidental arrival is paradoxically celebrated by the pervert's claim that he or she has arranged for the arrival of *this* stranger. In a world of unending surprises – of meetings with absolute strangers, often in foreign cities – the pervert covets the illusion that he or she has influenced the real to provide this exact sex object. The pervert is never to be surprised.

At the same time, although compelled to relieve the sexual excitation, and thus actually helpless in the face of the instinct, the pervert defies his or her state by over-identification with the nature of his or her instinctual life. If unable to prevail against the drive to be urinated upon, the pervert becomes an expert on urination and all sexual possibilities therein. He or she finds pornographic literature on the topic, discovers where fellow practitioners hang out, and keeps up with and often invents new types of equipment that elaborate the compulsion to new forms of expression. The pervert becomes master of that instinct, not its slave.

So the pervert masters two objects that have heretofore been devastatingly surprising: the object that arrives from the instinct (let's say, the wish to urinate on someone), and the other who comes from out of the real into the perverse zone to join in with the excitement before disappearing back into the real (like the other who meets the pervert in the wooded part of a park). Much more can be said about the pervert, but, by comparison with the hysteric, we hypothesise the pervert's character disturbance as his or her solution to flashes of maternal violence, which dissociate the pervert from his or her body, and which lead to intense mistrust of the other. The mother's use of his or her body for her own episodic sexual cathexes weds mother and child to excitation, even more bizarre, as it is partly generated by flashes of annihilation.

The hysteric's mother conveys her love of her infant through non-sexual means and indicates intense ambivalence towards the sexual body of the hysteric; the pervert's mother conveys flashes of sexual violence that drive the child's soul momentarily out of its body, as she cathects aspects of her infant's body as her sex thing. The hysteric represses his or her sexual contents to fulfil maternal desire; the pervert expresses his or her sexual contents to fulfil maternal desire. The hysteric sequesters sexual mental contents to assume innocence through transcendence; the pervert reveals sexual mental contents to assume decadence through self-debasement.

As Robert Stoller (1975) has emphasised, perversion is an erotic form of hate. As I imagine it, the pervert's externalisation of the instinctual process, whereby his or her inner compulsion must be linked to an actual other in a full-scale enactment of the sexual preoccupation, shadows the mother's rupture of the self's ordinary internality. It is as if the mother has slapped the infant with a look, jolting her child out of his or her unconscious and private renderings of instinctual processes, forcing her shocking presence upon the instinct-scheme as the origin of the instinct itself. Whereas ordinarily the instinct arrives from the self's nascent bodily states, choosing objects to structure and eliminate instinctual tensions (such as imagining water when thirsty), the pervert's instinct source seems derived from the shocking arrival of the other. Thus, adding to Freud's well-known phrase that the instinct is the demand upon the mind for work, we can say that in perversion, the instinct also expresses the demand upon the mind of the other for work. Instinct and other are fused, both demanding that the mind find a route for equivalent expressions.

The pervert's destiny is to accept this enforced link and transform it into his or her desire. The pervert is to take the disruption of the instinct and the shock of the other, and bind them into a sexual schema which can be repeated endlessly in his or her mind and which in practice will eventually make him or her prince/princess of his/her own darkness.

However messed up and bonkers the hysteric may seem, he or she is always loveable and loving. The pervert is eerie, with often toxic sexual excitements and strange acts of despair. Yet the pervert finds in his or her equally perverse partner true redemption: perpetrator or victim of hate, both partners feel that each has triumphed over cold violence itself, and out of this collaboration comes what Masud Khan (1983) terms a type of 'intimacy' that insists upon a familiarisation of the demilitarised zone that circumnavigates the maternal introject.

In assessing the pervert, the hysteric or the borderline, psychoanalysts can turn to their countertransferences to provide vital distinctions. The pervert and the hysteric, for example, can both be theatrical. How does one tell the difference between these two traits? Observation alone is unlikely to be determinative, as both the pervert and the hysteric also use theatres of the self for scopophilic purposes, and derive secondary gain from acting out. In listening to the account of the enacted, however, the psychoanalyst will have very different psychic matrices of response. The hysteric's theatre seems richly symbolic, always bringing associative responses to the psychoanalyst's mind, expressing a link between the hysteric's unconscious and the analyst. The pervert's theatre, although of interest and compelling, seems a terminal object and is not part of a signifying chain that either elicits or transmits latent unconscious contents. The psychoanalyst hearing the pervert's report of an enactment is unlikely to be moved by the account, which would suggest the arrival of unconscious associations.

A few words about being moved.

Freud's theory of technique is based entirely on the nature of the relationship between analysand and psychoanalyst. The patient is to free associate, especially reporting thoughts which seem irrelevant or unimportant, and the analyst is to enter a frame of mind – evenly suspended attentiveness – in which the analyst is not to concentrate on anything in particular, not to have expectations, not to remember anything in particular, 'and by these means to catch the drift of the patient's unconscious with his own unconscious' (Freud, 1923: 239). Practically speaking, in this frame of mind the psychoanalyst will be drifting inside the patient's material, and every so often will be struck by something. He or she will find a word, an image, a phrase, a person or an event described to be interesting. He or she will not know why it is interesting and this is, of course, exactly the point. The interest will be determined by the analyst's own unconscious as it links with the patient's unconscious. The analyst's craft, then, is on occasion – where appropriate – to echo the patient's word, image or description. So, if in describing an event in the afternoon when visiting a friend, for example, a patient says that he saw a helicopter travel overhead, and he pauses after this, and the analyst *feels* moved by this word/image, he or she will repeat it, simply saying 'helicopter?' If the analyst is in touch with the patient, unconsciously communicating with him, then this action will lead to immediate further associations. It will release more mental contents, which will naturally have been latent contents residing in this word/image. If the analyst has not been in touch with his patient, the material will fall flat, or the patient might even say, 'You want me to tell you about the helicopter?' – which of course indicates that the analyst's mirroring has been disruptive and unproductive.

Psychoanalysts at work with hysterics find themselves in unconscious communication with their analysands. With the rare exception of the acting-out malignant hysteric, the psychoanalyst finds that in his or her reveries he or she is moved by particular mental contents narrated by the patient, and when the analyst echoes them, the patient will respond by the production of further material. This collaboration is enormously important in the outcome of such an analysis, as the analysand is a creatively contributing psychic partner to the psychoanalysis, even if he or she is characterologically resistant. That is, even though the hysteric is motivated to remain a child who will never join the maturational process, in psychoanalysis he or she is an unconscious contributor to the analytical process itself, and in this way provides material that contributes to the analyst's effectiveness. In the countertransference, the psychoanalyst feels nourished by the patient, interested in the sessions, and senses that this session and others to follow are moving in lines of thought that will result in the occasional inspired idea occurring in the analyst that can lead to interpretation.

Psychoanalysts working with borderline patients do not feel this way. Borderline analysands can make manifest sense, such as describing events of the day before. But as Bion's theory allows, they have not subjected these experiences to a type of inner reverie, transforming them from beta (the undigested) into alpha (the digested). It is as if the unconscious has refused to engage the object world, even if it can record or photograph it. Indeed, instead of conveying knowledge about life or the self, borderline narratives seem to convey anti-knowledge, or what Bion terms –K. They reflect psychotic levels of thinking, which aim to break the link between psyche and reality, so that the mind can evade emotionally unacceptable recognitions. In the countertransference, the psychoanalyst feels somewhat suffused with anxiety; as though the patient, whilst not manifestly attacking the analytical process, is nonetheless engaged in insidiously destroying meaning. As discussed in earlier chapters, the borderline then very often bursts into intense prolonged rage where little that is said makes even manifest sense, and in this moment the borderline has conjured the unconscious primary object, which is the state of mental turbulence itself.

Psychoanalysts' countertransferences with all patients of course vary, according to other character aspects of the patient, and according to the particular character of the psychoanalyst. But there are striking similarities in the countertransferences of analysts working with borderline patients that allow us to make important distinctions of a diagnostic type with the hysteric. The analyst dreads the borderline. He or she looks forward to seeing the hysteric. The analyst's affective life with the borderline is a spectrum of anxiety: from low-level vigilance to outright terror. The analyst is fondly protective of the hysteric. The borderline totally lacks charm, humour and reparative grace, whilst the hysteric is well possessed of all three qualities.

The borderline's attack on links is a psychotic process that eliminates meaning, even if the borderline has a lot to talk about. Repression would seem to eliminate a link, but it is specific: it removes from consciousness a specific sexual mental content. Furthermore, as repression is intended to fail, derivatives of the missing link are always returning to consciousness in displaced form, both in the patient's narratives and, crucially, in the psychoanalyst's inner associations as well. Hysterics are unconsciously devoted to communicating themselves to the other, whereas borderlines seek malignant misunderstanding, because it is in the chaos of misalliance that they constitute the object of desire.

If an hysteric commits suicide in a psychiatric hospital, the staff grieve deeply. All seem to know that the hysteric has made a mistake, quite literally, since the hysteric has not understood what death is, and imagines being able to attend his or her own funeral. It seems such a terrible waste. Sadly, in a very different way, if the borderline commits suicide the clinical community has to deal with a very particular sense of guilt resulting from an uncomfortable sense of relief. The borderline suicide does not seem a waste of a life; on the contrary, one wonders how this person managed to live as long as he or she did.

The psychoanalyst working with the pervert is subjected to a type of unconscious communication driven by the patient. The pervert's description of sexual manifest events will be of interest, but its constituents will seem like isolated marks, unforgettable, yet not in themselves linking to further mental contents. The psychoanalyst, however, is not at a loss for thinking, but will usually find that he or she must work very hard to detect links between fragments of material in one hour and a previous hour, or an hour occurring weeks, if not months, before. The analytical container in this respect must actively gather the shards of meaning, which will not signify anything until that form of splitting which takes place in the pervert has been subjected to what we might think of as historical reverie on the part of the psychoanalyst. He or she must become an historian to the analysis, actively bearing the bits and pieces of mental material in mind, recurrently trying to revive his or her own unconscious, which will remain detached from the patient. The analyst, in other words, must find some form of life in an otherwise unconsciously lifeless world.

It is difficult to describe this accurately. The pervert is not uninteresting. His or her practices are often fascinating to think about. The pervert often lectures, rather than talks to, the analyst and yet his or her didactic style is also of interest, even if not moving. But the pervert has left his or her psyche-soma, the effect being that he or she is unconsciously cut off from the other. Where unconscious communication should be, there is stereotype. Where the hysteric speaks infinite variations on a single theme, enriching the analysis, the pervert speaks multiple themes with no variations. In time the psychoanalyst feels the pervert's discourse to become deadening, not unlike the reader's response to the cumulative effect of de Sade's *120 Days of Sodom*. However interesting it seems to be, at least initially, this is a work of almost deadening repetitiveness, curiously objectified by de Sade himself through his strange habit of repeatedly re-describing the main characters of the drama. It is as if he knows the reader will have a hard time remembering them. How strange. De Sade devotes what appears to be meticulous care in describing each character, yet they are not memorable in the least, so he attempts to make up for this by describing them again and again. Ironically, his re-descriptions add only to the overall deadening effect of what are intended to be unforgettable figures.

In the shadows of the pervert's repetitiveness is what Grotstein (1981) calls the 'background object', a mother who is not alive to the psychosomatic existence of her infant. Only in the occasional shock of her excitational use of her child, does she seemingly come alive. Out of the torpor of the pervert's ruminations seeps a kind of awful boredom, only now and then suspended by an intensely exciting acting out. The psychoanalyst in the countertransference will be 'rushed' out of inertness by the shock of a new-found sexual habit, or the threat of some risky acting out. This is a place where life can only be exciting, as once the excitement is gone, there seems to be no life at all.

Hysteria, perversion and the borderline, as categories of character breakdown, can be distinguished from one another within the psychoanalyst's countertransference, as the difference between the psychoneurotic, perverse and psychotic processes are profound. Hysterics can be frightening and paralysing, but even though the analyst may have a hard time thinking, such actions do not constitute the same attack on linking of which Bion writes. A great deal can be gleaned from a group's response to a clinical case presentation. Regardless of how mad the patient appears, if the group's response to the presentation is alive with ideas – interests, associations, links between contents, etc. – it is impossible for this to be a response to the borderline or perverse character. This is evidence, clinical evidence, of that kind of unconscious communication typical of the psychoneurotic personality. Alternatively, even if the presentation is full of seemingly interesting descriptions, if the group feels deadened by the presentation, with an overall sense of eerie emptiness, then this matrix suggests the patient is a pervert, even if as yet the case material does not manifestly point toward it. (The narcissistic personality has an emptying effect on the group, leaving it feeling sleepy, rather than deadened. The group also feels irritated, and aggressive towards the narcissist, which is rarely the case with the pervert.) If the group is fragmented, with its members having a hard time thinking, the observations in bits and pieces, and the overall effect one of anxiety and estrangement, this may be clinical evidence of the unconscious reception of a borderline personality.

Because the hysteric is gifted in identifying with and representing the desire of the other, it is imperative to keep in mind that the one figure whom they seek above all else to satisfy in the modern world is the psychoanalyst, the psychotherapist, the doctor or the holistic practitioner. Hysterics can successfully imitate schizophrenics, borderlines, narcissists and perverts. In determining diagnosis, then, two helpful factors are the psychoanalyst's countertransference and a group's response to a case report. Given that psychoanalysis became unusually invested in the concept of the borderline personality in the 1960s, it is especially important to take the clinician's manifest diagnosis of borderline with a pinch of salt. This could well be an hysteric, and one way of determining this would be to make the differential diagnosis discussed above from the countertransference.

Hysterics presenting themselves as other clinical objects of desire – such as a schizophrenic, for example – can also be detected by virtue of the presentation of (in this case) decidedly non-schizophrenic characteristics. Remember, they can produce all the symptoms of the schizophrenic, so it is no good saying that because the patient has auditory hallucinations, cannot distinguish between fantasy and reality, and has a thought disorder, this must be a schizophrenic. The hysteric can produce these symptoms. What one looks for are significant characteristics inconsistent with the schizophrenic, such as pleasure in secondary gain; a split-off observing part of the personality that takes some subtle pleasure in his or her enactments; a versatility of psychotic symptom presentation such as auditory, olfactory, somatic and visual hallucinations in a moving palimpsest, which would constitute an hysteric's movement within the psychotic identity; a capacity to move from very mad states of mind and behaviour to lucid, coherent and normal life; an ability when speaking to evoke associations in the other, which may be consciously registered by the other only in the sense that, whilst listening, it seems that the self is actually there, teasingly so.

While psychoanalysts in France usually follow Freud in comparing the hysteric to the pervert, psychoanalysts in other countries usually juxtapose the hysteric and the borderline. Space does not permit the kind of careful deconstruction of the history of this difference that it deserves, but I must take this up briefly. In 1974 Jean Laplanche, no doubt speaking on behalf of many French psychoanalysts, as reporter to an IPA (International Psychoanalytical Association) Congress panel on hysteria, protested against the 'desexualisation' of psychoanalysis, a protest which the French continue to lodge to the time of writing.

Indeed, it is arguable that the rise of the borderline personality in the 1950s, drawing psychoanalysts' interests towards the 'primitive' and the 'pre-oedipal', constituted an hysterical movement within the psychoanalytic community itself. It may well have been that psychoanalysis desexualised its own language and theories, announced through the signifier 'borderline', which then constituted a repression of the word 'hysteria'. From this moment on, psychoanalysis sought the hysteric in the name of the borderline. As hysterics seek to become the other's objects of desire, it may well be that they felt the analyst's desire for the borderline and presented the self as such long before the clinical community was celebrating this term.

Indeed, as Elaine Schowalter (1997) has argued in her brilliant book *Hystories*, hysteria is alive and well in the form of attention-deficit disorder, chronic-fatigue disorder, alien-abduction movements and the like. It is more than sad that the hysteric's capacity to fulfil the other's desire has meant that many people have dedicated their lives to romances with clinicians, presenting new 'sexy' diagnoses – such as multiple personality disorder – which inevitably earn accolades for the clinicians founding a new term or re-founding an old one, now rendered dramatically potent.

Yet, true to the nature of all intellectual movements, psychoanalysis progresses in 'swings and roundabouts', and in the early 1990s conferences on sexuality and hysteria sprang up, new and interesting books on hysteria were written, and psychoanalysis not only rediscovered hysteria, but may well also have recovered from its own forgetting.

So, finally, how do all the constituents of hysteria fall into the one integrated dynamic form promised in this book's introduction?

The hysteric specifies the body as the agent of his or her demise because its bio-logic brings sexual mental contents to mind. These ideas are repressed and/or converted to a body, which is silently loathed through mental indifference to it. The hysteric believes that sexuality destroys trust, a conviction that is cemented in the two great sexual epiphanies – at 3 and 13 – but this inclination has been communicated by the mother, who found the sexuality of her infant disturbing. The first repudiated pulsion of the infant is in the mother's mind, followed by her first conversion (from her repression of the infant's sexuality to the dead hand touching the genitals), which itself constitutes the first hysterical transmission. The mother offers reparation through a displaced erotisation, on to the non-genital erogenous zones of the body, and into her narratives and performances, where the child senses he or she lives as an alternative erotic object. The child unconsciously aims to enter the mother's imaginary and identify with and represent the self as the mother's object of desire. Of course, such explorations pick up all kinds of other internal objects, and a collateral fallout of such identification is the self's portrayal of others never known yet nonetheless taken into the self as part of its own imaginary. To be histrionic is to transfer the act of self envelopment to the other, to turn the self into the event that it senses itself to be inside, and to try to form the real into an imaginary. The hysteric would make of the entire world an auto-erotic scene, all the objects sexualised, yet with no binding genitality – just an endless sequela of foreplays, the only extinctions those of exhaustion and spent self states.

At any moment in time, therefore, the hysteric's psychic economy is over-determined by the body's insistence, experienced as divisive, inviting repression and conversion, on the one hand – to eliminate it – but, on the other, leading to histrionic self exhibitions which discharge the excitation through the theatre of the imaginary, which has momentarily enveloped the other into the auto-erotic fold. Conveying the image is marriage to the internal mother – the maker of images – and silent defiance of the symbolic order; words are used to paint pictures and to seduce the other into the dream world of the imaginary. Speaking, on the other hand, constantly returns the repressed mental contents, much to the chagrin of the hysteric, who becomes allergic to his or her own unconscious life. Hysterics enter the other (the analyst in the countertransference) as a charming child in adult form, seducing the other to be swayed by the image, seducing the other into abandonment of carnality and acceptance of transcendence to the higher orders of some divine presence, trying to destroy the other's participation in the maturational order that engages the self in the secular world.

The internal father is a shaky structure. Needing to adapt to reality – in order to fulfil the other's desire for socialisation – the hysteric hates a psychic structure that progressively separates the child from the open arms of the virgin mother. The maturational logic of the self – its destiny drive – is ambivalently regarded and true self realisations, through use of the object world, are retarded in order to signify loyalty to a past meant always to repudiate the future. Mother-past and father-future are a couple, the primal scene of which is intended to create a holy ghost in the present, who can magically move back and forth between maternal and paternal orders.

This is the picture.

As the reader will note, this dynamic – repression, conversion, indifference, transcendence, histrionics, transmission – is a complex that remembers the hysteric self's psychic history. No other character suffers this particular psychic history and no other character brings each of these constituents into this particular dynamic composition. Nor does any other character privilege virtually equal weight to the biological, psychic-developmental, object-relational, symbolic and cultural forces as does the hysteric – so much so that this character would appear crucified by their intersections.

It was not only the eastern Europeans who lived behind the iron curtain during the 1950s. With the hegemony of the term 'borderline', hysterics were shoved off the stage of psychoanalysis. Even though these performances were rightly seen as manifestations of their very conflict, it was far better that they be centres of attention than not, for their suffering is more complex than any other character who inhabits the world of the psychoanalytic imaginary. But with the *glasnost* of de-repression in 1990s psychoanalysis, we are likely to see the colourful garments of the hysteric return once again to our stage, there to clown around with us all, and to compel us to think them again and again.

Next time we think hysterics have disappeared, let's ensure someone asks after us, and calls for help.

References

Abraham, Karl. 'The ear and auditory passage as erotogenic zones', in *Selected Papers on Psycho-Analysis*. London: Maresfield Reprints, [1913] 1927, pp. 244–247.

Balint, Michael. *The Basic Fault*. London: Tavistock,1968.

Bollas, Christopher. *The Shadow of the Object*. London: Free Associations Books, 1985.

——. *Cracking Up*. New York: Hill & Wang, 1995.

——. *The Mystery of Things*. London: Routledge, 1999.

Breuer, J. and Freud, S. *Studies on Hysteria*, in *The Standard Edition of the Complete Psychological Works of Sigmund Freud*, Vol. 2. London: Hogarth Press and the Institute of Psycho-Analysis, [*S.E.* 2], 1895.

Chasseguet-Smirgel, Janine. *Creativity and Perversion*. London: Free Association Books, 1985.

Donnet, Jean-Luc and Green, André. *L'Enfant de Ca*. Paris: Les Editions de Minuit, 1973.

Fairbairn, W.R.D. 'The nature of hysterical states', in *From Instinct to Self*, ed. D. Scharff and E. Birtles, Vol. 1, 1994. pp. 13–40.

Ferenczi, Sándor. *Thalassa*. New York: *The Psychoanalytic Quarterly*, [1923] 1938.

Fletcher, John. 'Introduction: psychoanalysis and the question of the other', in Jean Laplanche, *Essays on Otherness*. London: Routledge, 1999, pp. 1–51.

Forrester, John. *The Seductions of Psychoanalysis*. Cambridge: Cambridge University Press, 1990.

Freud, Sigmund. 'On the Psychical Mechanism of Hysterical Phenomena: Preliminary Communication', in *Studies on Hysteria*, S.E. 2, 1895, pp. 3–17.

——. 'Fragment of an analysis of a case of hysteria', *S.E.*7, 1905a, pp. 7–122.

——. 'Three essays on the theory of sexuality', *S.E.* 7, 1905b, pp. 125–245.

——. 'My views on the part played by sexuality in the aetiology of the neuroses', *S.E.* 7, 1906, pp. 271–279.

——. 'Hysterical phantasies and their relation to bisexuality', *S.E.* 9, 1908, pp. 159–166.

——. 'Some general remarks on hysterical attacks', *S.E.* 9, 1909a, pp. 229–234

——. 'Analysis of a phobia in a five-year-old boy', *S.E.* 10, 1909b, pp. 3–149.

——. 'A note on the unconscious in psychoanalysis', *S.E.* 12, 1912, pp. 257–266.

—— 'On narcissism: an introduction', *S.E.*14, 1914, pp. 69–102.

—— 'The unconscious', *S.E.*14, 1915, pp. 161–215.

—— 'Mourning and melancholia', *S.E.*14, 1917, pp. 239–258.

——. 'A child is being beaten', *S.E.* 17, 1919, pp. 179–204.

——. 'Two encyclopaedia articles', *S.E.*18, 1923, pp. 235–259.

——. 'The dissolution of the Oedipus complex', *S.E.* 19, 1924, pp. 173–179.

——. 'Some psychical consequences of the anatomical distinction between the sexes', *S.E.* 19, 1925, pp. 243–258.

——. 'An outline of psychoanalysis', *S.E.* 23, 1940a, pp. 141–207.

Green, André. *Le Travail du Negatif.* Paris: Editions de Minuit, 1993.

——. 'The primordial mind and the work of the negative', *International Journal of Psycho-Analysis*, 79 (1998), pp. 649–665.

Grotstein, James. *Splitting and Projective Identification.* New York: Jason Aronson, 1981.

Khan, Masud. 1971. 'Infantile neurosis as a false-self organization', in *The Privacy of the Self.* London: Hogarth, 1974, pp. 219–233.

——. 'Intimacy, complicity and mutuality in perversions', in *Alienation in Perversions.* London: Hogarth Press, 1979, pp. 18–30.

——. 'Grudge and the hysteric', in *Hidden Selves.* London: Hogarth, 1983a, pp. 51–58.

——. 'None can speak his/her folly', in *Hidden Selves*, London: Hogarth, 1983b, pp. 59–87.

Kohon, Gregorio. 'Reflections on Dora: the case of hysteria', in *The British School of Psychoanalysis.* London: Free Association Books, 1986, pp. 362–380.

Kohut, Heinz. *The Analysis of the Self.* New York: International Universities Press, 1971.

Korfman, Sarah. *The Enigma of Woman.* Ithaca, NY: Cornell University Press, 1980.

Lacan, Jacques. *Ecrits.* London: Tavistock Publications, 1977.

Laplanche, Jean. *Seduction, Translation, Drives.* London: Institute of Contemporary Arts, 1992.

Lewis, C.S. *English Literature in the Sixteenth Century.* Oxford: Clarendon Press, 1944.

Lichtenstein, Heinz. 'Identity and Sexuality', in *The Dilemma of Human Identity*, New York: Jason Aronson, [1961] 1977, pp. 49–122.

Limentani, Adam. 'To the limits of male heterosexuality', in *Between Freud and Klein.* London: Free Association Books, 1989, pp. 191–203.

Mitchell, Juliet. 'Sexuality, psychoanalysis and social changes', *International Psychoanalysis*, 6, 1, (1997), pp. 28–29.

Modell, Arnold. 'Seminar', Beth Israel Hospital, Boston, 1973.

Muller, John P. *Beyond the Psychoanalytic Dyad.* New York and London: Routledge, 1996.

Phillips, Adam. 'Looking at Obstacles', in *On Kissing, Tickling and Being Bored.* Cambridge, MA: Harvard University Press, 1993, pp. 79–92.

Polanyi, Michael. *Personal Knowledge.* New York: Harper & Row, 1964.

Pontalis, J.-B. 'On death work', in *Frontiers in Psychoanalysis.* London: Hogarth Press, 1981, pp. 184–193.

Rosenfeld, Herbert. *Impasse and Interpretation.* London: Tavistock, 1987.

Ryle, Gilbert. *The Concept of Mind.* London: Penguin Books, 1963.

Scott, Clifford. 'Remembering Sleep and Dreams', *The International Review of Psycho-Analysis*, 2, (1975), 253–354.

Searle, John. *Expression and Meaning.* Cambridge: Cambridge University Press, 1985.

Schowalter, Elaine. *Hystories.* New York: Columbia University Press, 1997.

Steiner, John. *Psychic Retreats.* London and New York: Routledge, 1993.

Stewart, Harold. *Psychic Experience and Problems of Technique.* London: Routledge, 1992.

Stoller, Robert. *Perversion.* New York: Pantheon Books, 1975.

Wyatt, Sir Thomas. 'Description of the contrarious passions in a lover', in J. Hebel *et al.* (eds), *Tudor Poetry and Prose*. New York: Appleton-Century-Crofts, pp. 13–14.

Yarom, Nitza. *Body, Blood and Sexuality*. New York, San Francisco, Bern *et al.*: Peter Lang, 1992.

Index

Note: Where entries refer to footnotes the page number is followed by the footnote number, for example 97n1 refers to footnote number 1 on page 97.